Home Handbook

FIRST AID
& HOME SAFETY

Anne Charlish

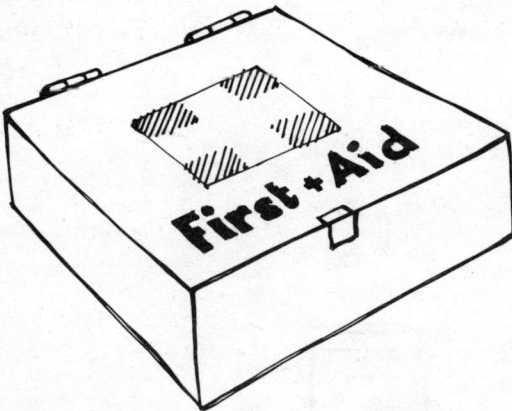

Ward Lock Limited · London

To Dr John Cutting for his patience and
affection and his concern for accuracy.

© Text & Illustrations Ward Lock Limited 1988

First published in Great Britain in 1988
by Ward Lock Limited, 8 Clifford Street,
London W1X 1RB, an Egmont Company.

Designed by Anita Ruddell

Illustrated by Paul Dewhurst

Text filmset in Baskerville No. 2
by MS Filmsetting Limited,
Frome, Somerset
Printed and bound in Great Britain
by Richard Clay Ltd, Bungay, Suffolk.

British Library Cataloguing in Publication Data

Charlish, Anne
 First aid and home safety.
 1. Residences. Safety
 I. Title
 363.1'375

 ISBN 0-7063-6652-2

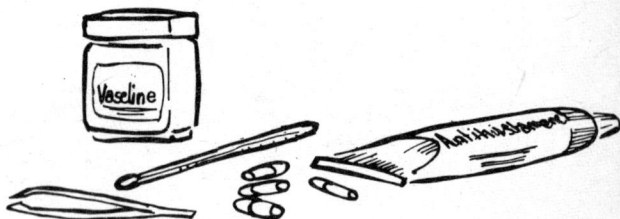

CONTENTS

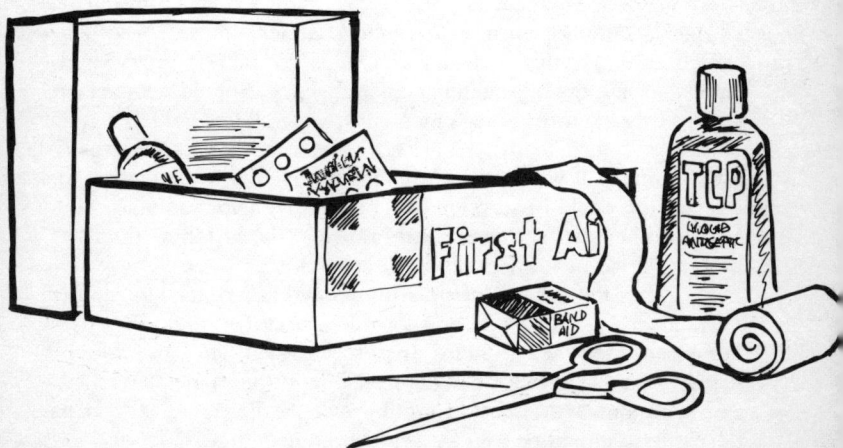

INTRODUCTION

First aid seems to many of us to be something that only enviably sensible and level-headed people can do: but there is no mystique in knowing what to do at the right time. Every one of us should be able to administer first aid treatments, particularly in a crisis when life may be at stake.

One in 3 of all accidents takes place in our own homes and the great majority of these are preventable. Chapter 1, therefore, is devoted to making your home as safe as it can be. Your next priority is to maintain a clean, well-stocked and comprehensive first aid kit in the house and a second in the car: these are described in Chapter 2.

One of the problems with serious accidents is knowing what to do first and knowing how potentially serious a casualty's condition may be. Chapter 3, then, is devoted to identifying quickly the sorts of conditions that require immediate qualified medical assistance, all of us should know when to dial 999 for an ambulance before doing anything else. Chapter 4 describes all the techniques for saving life in crucial circumstances, in which the casualty could die if you were unable to recognize the need for immediate action.

For genuine emergencies, such as, for example, when someone has stopped breathing or you suspect a heart attack, you will need to act straightaway. For this reason it is recommended that Chapters 3 and 4 be read at leisure and the information digested. Should you be faced with a truly life-threatening emergency, you will lose valuable, if not crucial, minutes if, firstly, you are not quite sure what *is* an emergency and, secondly, if you have to attempt to save life while reading the pages of this book. In addition, you may find it helpful to take a short course on first aid with your local branch of the St John Ambulance Brigade (listed in your telephone directory).

Part II of the book is intended to be used as a quick alphabetical reference to first aid treatments for minor accidents and ailments. A number of medical symptoms are also included here, for while not strictly treatable by first aid at home, it is important that you recognize such symptoms as prolonged vomiting, or a bleeding mole, as signs that the casualty should be seen by a doctor immediately.

· 1 ·

MAKING YOUR HOME SAFE

One in 3 of all accidents happens in the home, and the majority of these involve children. While all of us probably ought to know more about first aid than we do, making our homes safe and trying to prevent accidents happening should be our first consideration. If you have children or there's a possibility that children will visit your house, home safety is all the more important.

NOT WHAT IT SEEMS

When you look round your house critically, you may be surprised at just how much potential for accidents there is:

● The table lamp that looks perfectly stable – until it is knocked or pulled over.
● The wires to the stereo speakers that cross the carpet – just waiting for someone to trip over them.
● The table that looks solid – until you lean on one side.
● Glass-topped tables that may splinter under impact.
● A welcoming fire with no guard that may throw out hot sparks.
● A pretty rug on a polished floor with no non-slip backing grid.
● Mothballs, cleansers, sprays, medicines – all of which can deceive a child.

These are just some of the many danger spots illustrated in fig. 1, of which you should be aware.

THE BATHROOM

In Great Britain every year, some 26,000 accidents occur in the bathroom – in fact about 90 per cent of accidents involving electricity

Fig. 1

This diagram illustrates the most common risk areas in the house.
Those indicated by letters are hazards to watch out for continually.

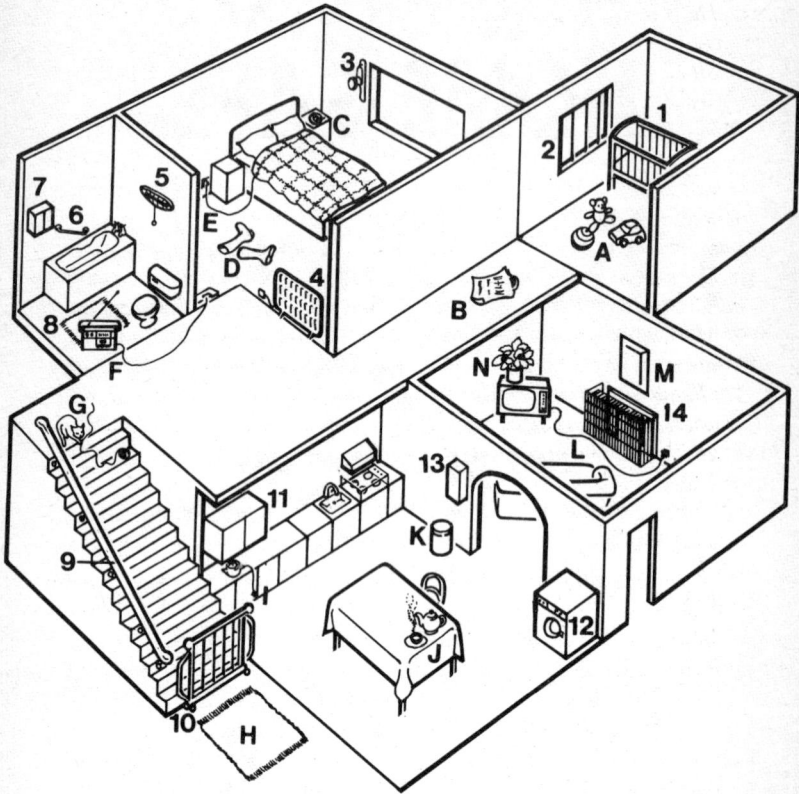

happen there. There are three chief hazards in the bathroom and they
are: water; water combined with electricity; and medicines.

□ **Taking a bath**

Bathing is the most likely time that something may go wrong. To avoid
falls grips set into the sides of the bath and a non-slip mat on its base are
essential, especially for young children and older adults. If your

Risk Areas

1. Don't put a pillow in a cot.
2. Put window bars in children's bedrooms.
3. Install a bedroom fire escape.
4. Have an enclosed heater rather than an open fire.
5. Set an electric heater high up on the wall. It should be controlled by a string-pull.
6. A hand-grip at the side of the bath prevents a fall.
7. Keep medicines in a cabinet, out of reach of children.
8. Use a non-slip bath mat to prevent falls.
9. Make sure the staircase handrail is safe.
10. Install safety gates at top and bottom to keep toddlers off the stairs.
11. Keep household chemicals in a cupboard away from children.
12. Fit a childproof lock on the washing machine.
13. Keep a fire blanket near at hand in the kitchen.
14. Stand a large fire guard in front of an open fire.

Hazards

A. Don't leave toys lying around – they can trip you up.
B. Don't leave plastic bags within easy reach of children.
C. Don't smoke in bed.
D. Don't leave footwear lying around to trip you up.
E. Don't have trailing flexes.
F. Don't introduce any mains-operated appliance into the bathroom.
G. Don't encourage pets to play on the stairs.
H. Don't have a slippery mat at the bottom of the stairs.
I. Don't leave flexes hanging down for children to reach.
J. Don't leave hot drinks on a table with an overhanging cloth if there are toddlers or small children around.
K. Don't have a rubbish bin that is easily accessible to toddlers.
L. Don't leave the television or the aerial plugged in at night, and don't have a trailing flex.
M. Don't hang a mirror or toys above a fire.
N. Don't put plants on the television – it is hazardous when you water them.

bathroom is tiled or lino covered, put a non-slip bathmat or cork mat on the floor.

When bathing a baby or young child, run the cold water first, followed by the hot to prevent the base of the bath becoming too hot. Test the temperature of the water before the child gets in to make sure that it is not much more than tepid to avoid discomfort and possible scalds. When you bath a child, be sure to give her your undivided attention: take the telephone off the hook; if the doorbell rings, either ignore it or take the child out of the bath and wrap her in a towel before you answer the door. A small child can drown in a bath easily and quickly while your attention is diverted for even, what you may consider to be, the shortest amount of time. Never take the risk.

When you take a bath yourself, avoid taking a very hot one late at night when you may be tired, and don't bath if you have drunk more alcohol than you usually do – you may doze off, and you could slip below the level of the water and drown.

☐ Incompatible partners

Water and electricity do not mix: the golden rule is that no one should be able to put one hand on or in water (or touch an appliance such as a lavatory) and, at the same time, be able to touch an electrical appliance or socket with the other. Electric lights should be controlled by string pulls within the bathroom and should be of a type recommended for bathrooms with the bulb and fitting completely enclosed. Any sockets (other than special shaving ones) should be located outside the bathroom. *Never* introduce an appliance, such as a hairdryer on an extension lead, into the bathroom. Fires should be set high up on the wall, well out of reach of children, and, again, should be controlled by a string pull.

☐ The medicine cabinet

This should be set high enough on the wall to be well out of reach of children, and ideally it should be lockable. All medicines – both prescription and over-the-counter – should be kept in their original containers and the labels left intact to avoid any confusion. Tablets and capsules can look like sweets to children, particularly if they are brightly coloured, so take care to store these away well out of reach. Always keep scissors and razors – and the spare blades – similarly safely stored.

☐ Keeping it clean

Bleach, lavatory cleansers and bath cleaners are all harmful if swallowed, and should be kept on a high shelf out of reach of children – not put away tidily in a cupboard beneath the basin where a toddler could decide to explore. At this age, remember, a child is infinitely curious.

THE KITCHEN

These days a kitchen is often the hub of a house, and you and your family may well spend more time there than anywhere else. And it is here that more home accidents happen than in any other part of the house: some 44,000 a year.

The most important principle to observe is that, as in the bathroom, water and electricity must be kept separate. All cables should be tucked away neatly with no trailing wires to trip up an unsuspecting child or adult. If you install new sockets, avoid placing them at skirting level: have them positioned at waist height if possible. Young children are extraordinarily curious as they explore the world around them and they will not yet appreciate that jamming a skewer or knife into an electric socket is dangerous. This can be prevented, however, by investing in socket covers to fix over any sockets which are not in use. If you have children, try to train them from as early an age as possible that sockets must not be touched.

☐ Things that need extra precautions

● Chipped glasses and cracked plates – throw them away.

● Plastic bags: store them safely in a high cupboard.

● Matches: keep these out of the sight and reach of children. If possible, use a gaslighter instead.

● Tablecloths: if you have children, put these away until they are older – a toddler could pull on them and bring down whatever is on top.

● Old furniture with flaking paint and splinters. All parents of young children should be aware that old furniture may be painted with lead-based paint which is toxic if sucked or eaten – strip it with a proprietary paint stripper in a well-ventilated area (preferably outdoors) and ensure any waste materials are safely disposed of.

● Electric iron: keep it in a cupboard; invest in a metal holder so that it can be put away while still warm. When ironing, always keep the ironing board close to the socket to avoid someone tripping up on trailing flex from the iron.

● Lamps with trailing cables: secure cables.

● Sharp objects such as knives, scissors, staples and any DIY tools: put them away safely. If you have children, do not keep your knives on a magnetic plate attached to the wall.

● A slippery floor: when it is washed, make sure everyone keeps clear until it is dry, or wash it while everyone is out.

● Oven: if you have children and you buy a new oven, make sure that the handle is childproof; otherwise, try to train a child that the oven, like electric sockets, is out of bounds.

☐ Safety in the kitchen: what you need

● Fire extinguisher.
● Fire blanket: to smother fat fires in frying pan or chip pan.
● Oven gloves: thick, sturdy ones with no frayed, bald patches.

☐ Preparing and cooking food

When you stand pans on the hob, always make sure that the handles are directed inwards, away from the front so that they do not protrude into the working area. If they do, a child could pull them or an adult could accidentally brush past them – with potentially dangerous consequences. This is especially true of large pans of boiling fat: in fact, when using chip pans, these are best placed on one of the back burners for safety.

If you should spill something – particularly on a tiled or lino-covered floor – mop it up straightaway and make sure that there is no residual grease which could cause a nasty fall.

Trolleys can be a problem with toddlers as they will tend to use them for support – which they cannot give.

STAIRS

All staircases should have firmly fixed handrails. If they become wobbly, this should be corrected without delay. Stair carpets should be firmly fixed, either with individual stair rods or with grippers all the way up the stairs on both sides. If you have just moved in, do not lay loose carpet; let the stairs remain bare until you have time to do the job properly.

The staircase should be well lit at all times with a light switch at both top and bottom, and should always be free of any objects that could trip someone up.

Take care if your dressing gown is full length; always have a free hand with which to raise the gown a little as you walk up or down. If your stair carpet is made of a synthetic material, you may find that vinyl-backed slippers will do just that – slip. Look for non-slip slippers with soles of cork, leather or sheepskin, for example, and replace them once they are shiny and worn. Alternatively, wear rubber-soled slippers or flip-flops. Beware your cat or dog on the stairs, and give them right of way!

Stairs present children of all ages with lots of fun – and their parents with problems. Older children love to play on them – sliding down banisters, and jumping four or more steps at a time – but you will have to discourage this unless you are prepared to deal with a broken arm or leg and many weeks of recovery. It is easier, with babies and toddlers, simply to restrict access to the stairs: invest in safety gates for both the top and the bottom of the stairs and never let the child practise any new skills of movement without supervision. The commonest accident that occurs on stairs happens when the confident toddler crawls up stairs, and then has no idea how to get down again . . . and falls. Such risks are not worth taking.

BEDROOMS

Choking and suffocation are the commonest forms of death in children under 5. For this reason, babies and young children should not be given pillows. Make certain that a child's cot is secure, that it has no rough edges, that a toddler cannot crawl right out of it, and that the rails at the sides are closely spaced. Blankets should be firmly tucked in at the sides of the bed or cot and the room well ventilated.

The windows of all bedrooms, or of any rooms from which there is a drop to the ground outside, should be properly secured with locks.

When buying night-clothes, check the label for an indication of low flammability.

☐ Electric blankets

When buying an electric blanket do ensure that it conforms to the British Standards Institution (BSI) safety standards. Look for the BEAB safety mark illustrated in fig. 2. Before using, do make sure that when you fit a 13-amp plug you only fit a 3-amp fuse.

The essential thing to remember when using electric blankets is that you must never use an under blanket on top or an over blanket

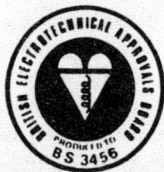

Fig. 2
The BEAB mark on an electric blanket indicates that it conforms to BSI safety regulations.

underneath. Always ensure that the under blanket is switched off and unplugged before getting into bed, unless of course you have an Extra Low Voltage (ELV) blanket. This is a specially manufactured under-blanket which can be left on all night – especially useful for elderly people. Over blankets can be left on, but if you do so, put nothing more than a light covering (e.g. a thin counterpane) over it.

All electric blankets should be serviced every second summer. Either contact the service department listed on the label sewn onto the blanket, or contact the BEAB.

THE LOFT

If you have a narrow stairway or ladder to the loft, make sure that they are perfectly safe and secure. If there are children around, invest in a childproof lock (not a simple bolt) for your loft to prevent a child exploring on his own. It is also well worth having a good light installed in the loft, and laying boards across the joists to prevent against potentially serious falls. Large DIY stores now supply packs of ready-cut sheeting suitable for laying in the loft.

FIRE

Fire is a potentially serious hazard in all areas of the home, and you should guard against this well.

All televisions should be unplugged at night and each aerial cable should be withdrawn from its wall socket, too.

Make sure that any cigarette butt is thoroughly extinguished in a proper ash tray. Never smoke in bed: you could doze off with a lighted cigarette in your hand. In fact smoking is so damaging to your own health, as well as to others, that you should stop altogether.

Frayed electrical cables or buzzing sockets should be dealt with as soon as they are noticed: both signify excessive wear and loss of insulating properties and therefore constitute a real risk of electrical fire. The electrical wiring system should be replaced, in fact, about every 20 years or so: if in doubt have a recommended electrician carry out a survey. Check for areas of rising or penetrating damp around sockets: this may result in electric shock when the socket is used. Electrical cables should either be properly cable-clipped to the skirting (not tucked beneath carpet) or concealed beneath furniture that is not usually moved (sofas, beds, chests and so on). Do not risk overloading the electrical circuit. This is caused by plugging too many appliances into one socket and could start a fire. If you are in any doubt about the combined electrical value of any of your appliances, consult your local electricity board showroom.

☐ **Smoke alarms**

It is wise to invest in a smoke alarm, placing it in the hall or at the bottom of the stairs. They are relatively inexpensive and can be installed by anyone with a screwdriver. Should a fire start downstairs, the alarm will react and will produce a loud beep that should wake you even if you are asleep. Do check it regularly as batteries do not last for ever.

FIRE DRILL

It is a good idea to work out the quickest escape route in the event of a fire occurring in various parts of the house. Organize your family and practise this occasionally. If a fire should start:

● Your priority is to get you and your family out as quickly and calmly as possible and dial 999 for the fire service.

● If the fire is confined to one area, such as a flaming chip pan on the kitchen hob, smother the pan with your fire blanket. Do *not* immerse the pan in water. Do not prejudice your chances of escape by trying to fight the fire.

● Do not ever attempt to put out a fire, or the smouldering start of one, involving foam-filled sofas and armchairs. The fumes that are given off are highly toxic and can kill in minutes.

● If the fire starts downstairs at night and you are upstairs, quickly put on dressing gown and slippers and pick up the nearest thing to hand to wrap around your head (towel or thick jersey, for example). Do not pick up anything else *whatsoever*. Speed is of the essence: you cannot know whether there will be a gas explosion, fumes given off by smouldering furniture foam or flames creeping up the stairs. If you have to walk through a room of intense heat, your dressing gown, slippers and head wrap will protect you. Should any of these catch fire, you will be able to throw these protective items off quickly once you get outside.

● If you have to go through a smoke-filled area to safety, crouch down low (as heat rises, the closer to the floor you are, the cooler the temperature).

See also Asphyxia in Part II.

OUT AND ABOUT

☐ In the garden

Some 250,000 people in Great Britain need hospital treatment each year as a result of an accident in the garden.

When mowing the grass, check first that children and pets are well away from the area. If your mower has an electrical cable, be extra vigilant at all times to ensure the cable does not become entangled in the motor; and keep your feet and your hands well clear of the cutting edge.

All garden tools and implements should be put away tidily in a shed or garage; if you don't have one, build a lean-to with corrugated iron.

Take special care with weedkillers, fertilizers, pesticides, insecticides and, indeed, anything that, if a young child puts it into her mouth, could prove fatal. Never decant any highly poisonous substances into an innocent-looking bottle such as a milk bottle or orange squash bottle; and keep all such products on a high shelf out of reach of any children.

Fencing and gates should be kept in good repair (and, if you have children, properly secured) and paved areas should be kept free of moss and wet leaves to reduce the likelihood of falls.

If you have a pool of any description, even a shallow plastic paddling pool, *always* stay with a child and *always* empty it after use, both to guard against a drowning accident and to prevent a child or a pet drinking water that may well be contaminated. Keep children well away from bonfires, barbecues and firework displays. Do not let children eat freely from the garden, and extend this rule to the countryside as well: berries, mushrooms and toadstools are for the *expert* adult only.

☐ In the country

With natural beauty come natural hazards, too, and these may come as a surprise to the city dweller. Make sure that both you and any children with you can tell the difference between a cow and a bull – never enter a field containing a bull.

Never walk too close round the back of a horse as it may kick out just to make sure it's not going to be attacked from the rear. Barbed wire is usually intended to keep animals in and humans out – with good reason. Don't try to crawl through, and if you should open a gate to walk round (not across) a field, be sure to shut it after you. Treat geese and swans with respect at all times, and always be extra careful with all animals during the nesting and breeding season. Take care as you explore streams and rivers and avoid damp, boggy areas.

☐ **On the beach**

Sun and water are both powerful natural hazards on their own and, in combination, they are even more dangerous. When you are sunbathing at the beginning of the season and your skin is delicate after being covered all winter, make sure that you use a good sun-protection cream with the appropriate screening factor for your skin. Never doze off in the hot sun. If it is very hot, babies and young children should always wear a hat for the middle 3 hours of the day.

If you swim, towel yourself when you come out and re-apply the sun-protection cream. The salt in the water makes it more likely that you will become sunburned.

Skin cancer can develop as a consequence of too long an exposure to hot sun, so moderation is the key.

The seaside is great fun for children, but never forget that the sea can be a killer and that the risk of drowning is ever present. Never, ever let young children swim unattended or get out of their depth. Never let them float on lilos or dinghies without you close by in the water: a sudden, strong breeze could take them quite a way out. Lastly, beware yourself of strong currents and always heed notices warning you that it is unsafe to swim.

☐ **Safety at sport**

Whatever sport you enjoy, make sure that you wear the correct headwear and footwear and that you are taught professionally the techniques of a game or sport. This is particularly important in skiing, riding, golf and squash, and for the perilous activities of hang gliding, water skiing, parachuting and windsurfing.

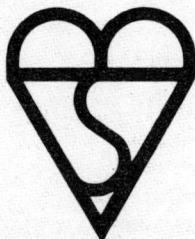

Fig. 3
The kite mark on a product indicates that it conforms with the BSI standard of quality.

Skiers Make sure your boots are a good fit. These must be attached to the skis by a professional and the pressure release mechanism carefully checked. Do not ski off piste without a recommended, experienced guide. *Always* wear ski goggles when skiing: these should be made of unbreakable glass and they can be made to your own prescription.

Riders Don't exceed your own capability or that of the horse. Never attempt a jump that *you* fear is too high, and don't urge the horse to do something *it* senses is potentially dangerous.

Safety at home and at leisure is largely a matter of common sense and being observant: if you reduce the hazards *and* if you're lucky, you should never have to use emergency first aid measures and only rarely the simplest of first aid techniques.

POISONOUS SUBSTANCES

You may be surprised at the large number of potentially lethal substances in your home. While an adult would not think of imbibing most of the items in the following table, a child could well do. To a child a mothball looks like a sweet, cough syrup and nail varnish resemble fruit drinks, and bleach could be water. The following table is a comprehensive list of both common and less common household poisons which, if children are around, should be kept well out of reach.

Should you suspect a case of poisoning, call for an ambulance first (dial 999) and then run down the list quickly to determine the possibility of the casualty having had access to any of these poisons.

NOTE In children under the age of 10, 4 out of 5 deaths by poisoning are caused by drugs taken accidentally without supervision; and in nearly one-quarter of these drug-induced poisoning deaths, aspirin was the cause. No child under the age of 12 should be given aspirin or anything containing aspirin, because of its newly discovered association with Rey's Syndrome.

What is poisonous?

alcohol, even in small quantities in the case of children
aspirin in large doses
Atropa belladonna (deadly nightshade)
barbiturates
belladonna (deadly nightshade)
benzodiazepines
berries, from many species
bleach

carbon monoxide
car exhaust fumes (carbon monoxide)
caustic soda (soda crystals)
cough syrup, do not exceed stated dose
deadly nightshade
***Digitalis** (foxglove)
dry cleaning solvents
Epsom salts in large quantities
food, if contaminated
foxglove (Digitalis)
fungi, many species
***holly**
household cleaners
illegal drugs, including opium, heroin, cocaine, crack, amphetamines
insecticides
insect stings
iodine
***laburnum**
lead (notably in the form of lead paint, pencils, and around leaded windows)

lighter fuel
matches
mothballs
mushrooms, many species (other than the variety bought)
nail varnish
nail varnish remover
paracetamol
paraquat
perfume
phosphorus (from matches, etc.)
plasticine
shoe creams and polishes
slug pellets
snake bites
tobacco
turpentine
vitamins A and D in large doses
weedkiller
white spirit
wood preservative treatments
***yew**

*Apart from the five most common poisonous plants listed above, there are many, many others. Many fungi, too, can prove fatal. It is wise not to eat anything, and to discourage a child from doing so, while in the garden or out on country walks.

YOUR
FIRST AID KIT

First aid is literally the first help you can give to an injured person, and that help should be given as quickly and as efficiently as possible. Because of this, it is vital that your first aid kit should contain everything you need and be readily to hand when an emergency occurs.

You can buy a first aid box; alternatively, you can use a biscuit tin that is completely clean. Label it clearly, and always keep it in the same place so that everyone knows where it is, making sure that it is out of the reach of young children. If you have a car, you should keep a duplicate kit in it at all times – do not be tempted to leave it in the garage because its rattling irritates you. Wrap it or attach it with sticky tape to a shelf in the car or fix it similarly in the boot.

WHAT SHOULD IT CONTAIN?

Your first aid kit should contain:

- antiseptic solution such as Dettol or TCP
- antiseptic cream such as Savlon
- Vaseline
- antihistamine cream for stings
- calamine lotion for irritating skin conditions
- iodine
- oil of cloves to relieve toothache
- surgical spirit to clean instruments
- eyebath, eye-cleansing liquid and eye pads
- soluble aspirin (for adults only)
- paracetamol for children (liquid for children under 6)
- lipsalve
- thermometer
- scissors

- tweezers
- safety pins
- plasters in various sizes and shapes
- adhesive dressings: 1 roll of adhesive dressing strip and 2 or 3 packs of perforated film adhesive dressings
- prepared sterile dressings in various sizes
- cotton wool: 1 roll
- crêpe bandages in three widths
- gauze: 1 roll
- elastic ankle bandage
- triangular bandages
- sling
- paper tissues
- a small hand mirror (to check for breathing)
- comprehensive and illustrated first aid book

▲ *Your First Aid Kit*

☐ **In the car**

All the items that you keep in your first aid kit at home will prove useful. You will also certainly need bigger bandages, dressings and gauze with which to staunch bleeding in the event of a traffic accident. A warm blanket is a good idea.

There are a few other items that, although not part of a first aid kit, may prove invaluable for your safety. A large torch, a fire extinguisher and red warning triangle (compulsory in some countries) will all be useful in the event of an emergency. Finally, your car should contain a spare wheel in good condition and with the correct inflation, a set of tools for basic repairs, and a pencil and paper.

Most people tend to ensure that their car contains all these things only when they are about to go on long journeys or on holiday. However, the majority of accidents occur within 2 miles of home. Statistically, therefore, you are more likely to need your first aid kit on a quick trip to the shops than you are on an annual holiday.

MAINTAINING YOUR KIT

The importance of replacing the items in your first aid kits really cannot be over emphasized. Even if you use only one sterile dressing in a pack, throw the rest away for they will no longer be sterile. Make sure that everything is thoroughly hygienic and ready for immediate use: the thermometer, for example, should be shaken down and washed in an antiseptic solution after each use.

·3·

KNOWING WHEN TO GET HELP

First aid can save life, it is true, but it is also essential to be aware of those instances in which it is crucial to obtain qualified medical assistance as soon as possible. This chapter, then, is designed to encourage and enhance your own instincts of common sense; it is not intended to be used as a quick reference in an emergency. Emergency measures – that is, the techniques that you will have to use in an emergency situation – are detailed in the next chapter. You should also refer to the appropriate entry in Part II, which describes the first aid and emergency treatments for all common conditions and symptoms, listed in alphabetical order from 'asphyxia' to 'winding'.

EMERGENCY SITUATIONS

If you encounter a casualty with any of the following conditions, you will know that some action is required from you straightaway. You will also require, for all these conditions, emergency medical assistance. Either dial 999 for an ambulance, or summon a doctor (in some rural areas, this may be quicker than an ambulance). If there is no other helper present, administer appropriate first aid and then seek professional help.

- suspected broken bone
- conscious but pale, limp, silent
- bleeding profusely
- unable to move
- difficulty in breathing, as in asthma attack or choking
- no longer breathing

- rescued from the water (inert, silent)
- unconscious
- starting to give birth

☐ Suspected broken bone

If possible relieve any pressure on the affected area. If the pain is thought to be in or near the spine, do not make any attempt in any circumstances to move the sufferer. If you move someone with a back injury, you are taking the serious risk of further damaging the spine and this could lead to permanent paralysis. They must be kept warm and an ambulance called without delay.

☐ Conscious but pale, limp and silent

The casualty may be in shock; *see* Chapter 3, page 25, for treatment. Keep the person warm, and do not give anything to eat or drink; you should call for emergency assistance. If the person has suddenly become pale and limp for no obvious reason, take the pulse (*see* Chapter 4, page 30). If it is slow and weak, call for help and prepare to give the kiss of life and heart massage if necessary (*see* Chapter 4, pages 30–35). If the person was already ill but seems to be worsening, call for a doctor.

☐ Bleeding profusely

First, try to staunch the bleeding (*see* Chapter 4, pages 36–37). Any severe bleeding is serious, but if the blood appears to be spurting from the body, you will know that an artery has been cut, and emergency assistance is vital. Use a sterile dressing if possible, but if someone is bleeding very severely, it no longer matters whether the dressing is sterile or not; the blood loss must be slowed. Apply pressure to the wound, elevate it if you can, and try to keep the edges together if possible, while you seek hospital treatment.

☐ Unable to move

If someone complains that they are unable to move with or without pain in the back, make sure that they are warm but do not attempt under any circumstances to move them. Call for an ambulance.

If they are unable to move because of pain in either leg, help them to a comfortable position, keep them warm and call for an ambulance.

▲ *Knowing When to Get Help*

☐ **Unconscious**

Make sure first that the person is still breathing (*see* Chapter 4). If they are not, give them the kiss of life and heart massage straightaway. If they are, loosen any clothing around the neck and make sure that the area is well ventilated; then place them in the recovery position (*see* Chapter 4, pages 35–36) and make sure that they are warm. If it is a simple faint, they will come round within a minute or two. If they do not come round quite quickly, call for an ambulance. If you know that the person is diabetic, you should suspect diabetic coma (*see* Part II). If the person has had an epileptic seizure, it may take some time for them to come round.

☐ **Difficulty in breathing**

If the cause is clear – for example, the person is choking – treat accordingly (*see* Chapter 4, page 39). If there is no obvious cause, call for an ambulance, loosen any restrictive clothing around the neck, seat the person comfortably and try to get them to slow their breathing rather than quicken it in response to panic.

☐ **No longer breathing**

Perform the kiss of life and heart massage immediately (*see* Chapter 4).

☐ **Rescued from the water**

If the person is unconscious, treat as above.

☐ **Starting to give birth**

Some women deliver a baby within 20 minutes of the first signs, while others may take as long as 36 hours or more. For this reason, if you find yourself in the position of helping someone in labour, you need to determine whether you have time to help the woman get to hospital or whether you should offer immediate assistance. If the contractions are coming every couple of minutes and the woman tells you that she can feel the baby's head emerging, you may well not have time to reach the hospital, and you should prepare to help (*see* Part II).

QUICK TESTS

All the above are instances in which life may be at stake if you fail to take the appropriate action. Some cases may not be so clear cut,

---

however. If, from your observations, you are not sure how serious the case is, there are a number of simple tests you can do to help you judge.

☐ Check breathing

Watch for any sign of breathing, such as the chest and abdomen rising. Place your ear to the casualty's chest and listen for the sound of breath being drawn, or put your face close to the casualty's mouth to see if you can feel their breath on your cheek. If you are still not sure whether the person is breathing or not, take the pulse and/or hold a mirror to his mouth. If the mirror does not steam up, you should assume that he is not breathing.

☐ Pallor

A deathly white or greenish white pallor is a good indication of something seriously wrong. So, too, is a greyish or bluish pallor.

☐ Temperature

If the cause of ill health is not evident but was clearly not caused by a sudden accident, then take the temperature. Place the thermometer beneath the tongue, or in the case of a young child, beneath the armpit. Leave for 2 minutes before removing. If it is over 104°F (40°C), or under 95°F (35°C), life may be at stake, and you must ensure that a doctor is coming or otherwise call for an ambulance. When you call a doctor, be sure to tell him or her of the temperature reading and any other symptoms.

EMERGENCY OR NOT?

Some emergency situations do not present themselves so dramatically but may nevertheless represent a threat to life. With these, you cannot afford to rely upon instinct or the simple tests outlined above to judge whether to seek immediate professional help.

☐ Chest pain

This could be indigestion but it could equally be a heart attack. If the person is over 40 and fighting for breath, it could well be the latter, but in a teenager, it is more likely to be indigestion or over exertion.

▶ *Knowing When to Get Help*

☐ Acute and/or prolonged abdominal pain

You should seek professional assistance immediately as this could be the first outward sign of a number of acute and serious conditions.

☐ Poisoning

Whenever poisoning is suspected, call for an ambulance immediately or take the person straight to your nearest casualty department, whichever is quickest. Do not wait and see: it is better to act quickly to prevent the possibility of internal damage.

☐ Animal bites

Common sense can help you here: if your own dog gives you a playful nip and does not break the skin, there is not much to worry about. However, if a strange dog bites you severely and draws blood, you should go to your nearest casualty department without delay. Snake bites and parrot bites should always be treated as an emergency as well.

☐ Chemical burns and splashes

Chemical burns and splashes of any such substance, especially in the eyes, should be dealt with in hospital. If in doubt, telephone first. Some chemicals, such as wood preservative treatments, can be washed off the skin in the event of small splashes. Large quantities, however, are more potentially dangerous for the substance can penetrate the skin and continue to be active, irrespective of thorough cleansing of the skin's surface.

☐ Cuts and wounds

You may clean and dress these yourself, but you should also take the person to your nearest casualty department if you observe any of the following:

● The cut is deep and there is either earth or manure in or near it. A tetanus vaccination will probably be given.
● Bleeding is heavy.
● The wound looks too open to be able to heal naturally, thus requiring stitches.
● A facial cut that is deep, particularly if it is near an eye or the mouth.

Because the facial area moves constantly, thus preventing rapid healing, these cuts often require stitches to ensure the wound heals neatly.

□ **Severe chill**

If someone is severely cold to the touch, behaves irrationally, has difficulty in moving and speaking and has a subnormal temperature, you should suspect a chill so severe as to be classified as hypothermia, a very serious condition (*see* Part II).

□ **Shock**

If someone suffers an injury or illness they may experience what is known as traumatic shock. In medical terms, this refers to the weakened condition, which can vary from faintness to complete collapse that results from lack of blood supply or body fluid. Symptoms include paleness, cold clammy skin, rapid pulse, fast shallow breathing, shaking, restlessness and anxiety, and thirst.

1 Lay the casualty down. Turn her head to one side and raise her feet (unless a fracture to the lower body is suspected).
2 Cover her loosely with a blanket or coat and loosen any restrictive clothing.
3 Call for urgent medical help.
4 If the casualty complains of thirst, moisten her lips with water: do not let her drink. Monitor her breathing and be prepared to resuscitate if necessary.

▲ *Knowing When to Get Help*

CHILDHOOD ILLNESSES

Babies and children tend to fall ill quite dramatically, often with high temperatures and their condition worsening more quickly than you would expect in an adult. Always call a doctor in such cases. Nine times out of 10 he or she will diagnose one of the straightforward childhood illnesses (*see table overleaf*).

There is no need to be alarmed when one of these normal illnesses occurs in your child. It is far better that they suffer them now rather than in later years, as many of them tend to be more severe in adults than in children. For example, mumps can be a very painful illness as an adult and, in rare cases, can permanently damage or destroy a man's fertility.

Illness	Symptoms	Incubation	Treatment	Prevention
Measles	Raised temperature, dry cough, red eyes and runny nose. Spots appear inside mouth on about 3rd day, although temperature drops. On 4th or 5th day, temperature rises again and rash appears on body, trunk first, then limbs.	7–14 days. Disease is usually over within a week of symptoms appearing.	Sponge patient with tepid water to reduce temperature. Be alert to the possibility of complications; call doctor in case of earache or headache.	Inoculation.
Chickenpox	Extremely itchy blisters, together with raised temperature and headache.	7–21 days. Children usually recover within 10 days of symptoms appearing.	Apply calamine lotion to the spots and blisters and prevent the child scratching them.	None.
Mumps	Glands at side of face and below ears swell. Swallowing may be painful. Testes and ovaries may become swollen and inflamed.	14–28 days. Still infectious for 7 days after swelling goes down.	Give lots of liquids and puréed food if swallowing is painful.	None.

Rubella (German measles)	Raised temperature; swollen glands; slight rash on 1st or 2nd day, first on face and then on body for day or two. May produce no obvious symptoms.	14–21 days. Symptoms disappear 4 or 5 days after onset.	None for this mild disease in children but do not allow any pregnant woman to be in contact with your child. (Do not take them to the doctor's surgery for this reason.)	Inoculation for girls between 11 and 14.
Scarlet fever	High temperature, sore throat, furry tongue. Rash on 2nd day on face, covering rest of body and limbs by 3rd day. Rash fades, giving way to peeling, which may go on for another 14 days.	1–7 days.	Tepid sponging to reduce temperature.	None.
Glandular fever	Similar to 'flu: headache, fever, sore throat, malaise. Also swollen glands in neck, armpits and groin.	Major symptoms clear within 2–3 weeks but feeling of lethargy and depression may persist.	Plenty of liquids, plus rest. Be alert for complications such as jaundice, and rash like that of rubella.	None.

▲ *Knowing When to Get Help*

The remaining childhood illnesses of *diphtheria, pertussis (whooping cough), tetanus* and *polio* are all prevented by the DTP or triple vaccine and polio vaccine given at 3 months, 5–6 months and 9–11 months. Vaccination against diphtheria and polio is given to children again when they start school (and polio vaccination again at 16–18 years); tetanus vaccination should be repeated at 5-yearly intervals.

Many parents worry about administering the whooping cough vaccine because of the small risk of brain damage. The risk of death or brain damage following whooping cough itself, however, is many times greater than that resulting from immunization. No child should be given whooping cough vaccine if they have had seizures ('fits') or if there is a family history of them. A child should not be given a second dose of the vaccine if she or he has a fever or has had any severe local or general reaction to the first dose, for example, convulsion, shock or high-pitched crying. Protection can still be given against diphtheria, tetanus and polio.

·4·

EMERGENCY MEASURES

You are suddenly faced with an extreme emergency. What should you do?

There are seven techniques considered essential for saving life:

- the 'kiss of life', otherwise known as mouth-to-mouth/nose respiration or mouth-to-mouth/nose ventilation
- chest compression, also known as heart massage
- the recovery position (said by some experts to be the single most important technique)
- staunching severe bleeding
- abdominal thrust, also known as the Heimlich manoeuvre
- life-saving in water
- alternative method of artificial respiration

All of these, in one way or another, involve the ABC of saving life:

- ☐ A for airway
- ☐ B for breathing
- ☐ C for circulation

These are the principles of saving life and should be an automatic response. Is the airway clear so that the person can breathe? Is their chest rising and falling, indicating that they are breathing? Is their heart beating?

Before any emergency measure can be carried out, it is important to know how to find out whether a person is breathing and if their heart is beating.

☐ Check breathing

First of all, simply observe: watch for any sign of breathing, such as the chest and abdomen rising and falling. You can also place your ear to the casualty's chest and listen for the sound of breath being drawn, or you can put your face close to that of the person and see if you can feel their breath on your cheek. If you have a small mirror readily at hand, you can check to see if it becomes steamed up with breath.

☐ **Check pulse**

To find out whether the heart has stopped beating the pulse must be taken. The most common site for taking this is the wrist, by placing the tips of 3 fingers on the inside of the arm on the thumb side. In an emergency, however, it is more reliable to take the pulse at the neck. Place your finger tips in the hollow between the voice box and the adjoining muscle. If there is no pulse begin heart compression immediately.

THE KISS OF LIFE

If a person has stopped breathing, you must give him the kiss of life immediately.

1   Place the person face up on the ground if possible. If this is not possible – say, he is slumped over the wheel of a car or over a desk and is too heavy to move – move his head backwards. In either case, the chin should be pointing upwards.

2   Turn the face quickly to one side and, using your index and middle fingers, remove any obvious foreign matter (including false teeth if they are blocking the airway) from the mouth.

3   Place one hand under the person's neck and, with the other, press down on his forehead so that his neck is arched and his chin tilts upwards with the mouth open (fig. 4). This will ensure that the tongue is lifted back to clear the airway. Remove the hand from under the neck and, using finger and thumb, squeeze the nostrils so that no air can escape.

4   Now take a deep breath, open your mouth as wide as possible and place it on the casualty's, completely sealing it (fig. 5). (If you can't get to the casualty's mouth properly, squeeze the lips shut with your thumb and perform mouth-to-nose resuscitation instead, blowing your breath into the casualty's nostrils.) Blow out steadily. As you do this, look to see if the casualty's chest rises, indicating that he is breathing.

5   Once you see the chest rise and fall, you will know that you have succeeded in getting air into the casualty's lungs. Now give another breath, and release your mouth momentarily (fig. 6).

Fig. 4

Support the neck with one hand and press down on the forehead with the other hand to tilt the chin up and the head back.

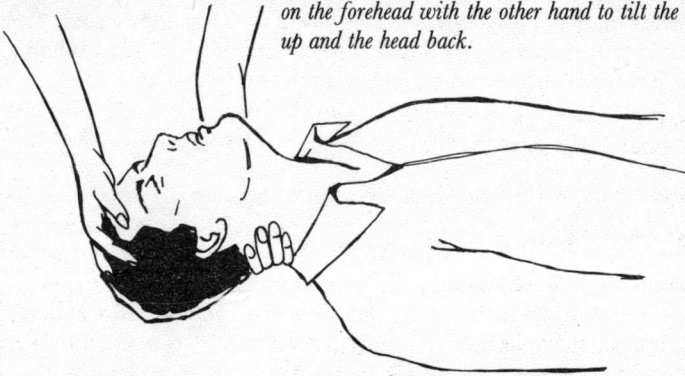

Fig. 5

Take a deep breath and place your mouth on the casualty's, completely sealing it. Breathe out steadily.

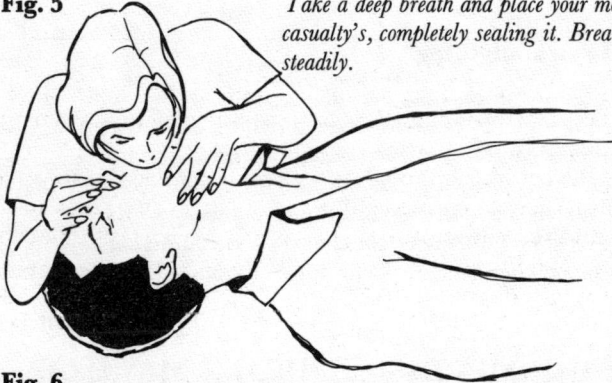

Fig. 6

Once you see the chest rise and fall, give another breath and release your mouth momentarily.

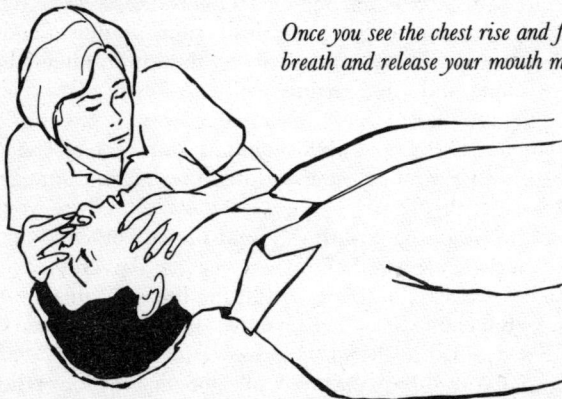

▲ *Emergency Measures*

6 After you have given 4 or 5 breaths, check the pulse. If it is not present, you must also give chest compression (*see below*). If the heart is beating, continue with the kiss of life, timing your breaths by the natural rise and fall of the casualty's chest.

7 Don't give up. Twenty minutes or even longer may seem like an eternity in this situation, but it may very well represent the difference between life and death.

□ Giving a baby the kiss of life

You will probably find that, as an infant's mouth is so small, you will need to give mouth-to-mouth-and-nose resuscitation rather than mouth-to-mouth. Place your mouth over the baby's mouth and nose and proceed as above, remembering to blow out very gently.

□ Will I catch anything?

Yes, you may if the casualty is suffering from an infectious illness. However, the chances of contracting anything life-threatening are very slim indeed, and it is safe to concentrate on saving life.

Although the AIDS virus has been found in saliva in very small quantities, no one has ever caught the virus in this way. AIDS is still a very rare disease and, therefore, the chances of encountering a casualty who may be on the verge of death but is also an AIDS carrier are remote.

CHEST COMPRESSION (HEART MASSAGE)

If the heart has stopped beating and you are therefore unable to detect any pulse, act immediately to get it beating again, so that blood continues to circulate around the body and reaches the brain, thus avoiding the possibility of brain damage.

You will need to perform this technique together with the kiss of life: if there are two of you, one should perform mouth-to-mouth resuscitation while the other carries out chest compressions. Alternate tasks every few minutes.

1 Lay the casualty on his back with the head tipped back and the chin pointing upwards. Kneel beside him, facing the chest (*see diagram*). Locate the breastbone (sternum) in the centre of the chest and find its lower end, where the ribs meet at its base. Place the heel of your hand along the breastbone and position it about 2.5–3 cm (1–1½ in) up from the base. Check the position by locating the top of the breastbone between the 2 collar bones (extending outwards from the base of the neck towards the shoulders) and the bottom of the breastbone where the 2 bottom ribs meet. You should aim to put your hand about halfway up the lower half of the breastbone.

2 Place the heel of your other hand upon the first and interlock your fingers, making sure that they do not dig into the casualty's chest as you start to exert pressure (fig. 7).

3 Lean forward so that your head and shoulders are directly above the casualty's chest. Keeping your elbows straight, push firmly and steadily on the breastbone until it descends about 4 cm ($1\frac{1}{2}$ in) towards the spine. Release the pressure immediately and repeat (fig. 8).

4 You will need to compress the chest 15 times, at a rate of some 80 times a minute (15 compressions should take just over 11 seconds).

Fig. 7

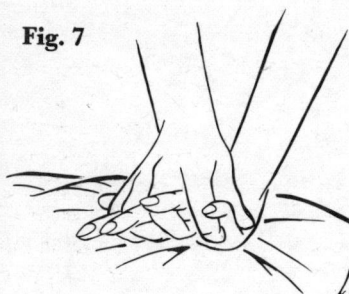

Place the heel of one hand along the breastbone. Put your other hand on top and interlock your fingers.

Fig. 8
Keeping your elbows straight, press firmly on the breastbone, compressing the chest by about 4 cm ($1\frac{1}{2}$in). Release and then repeat.

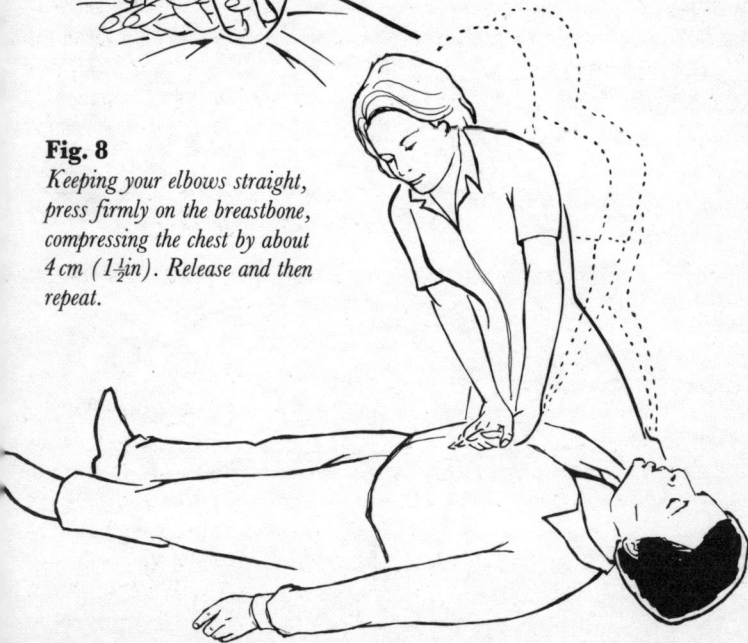

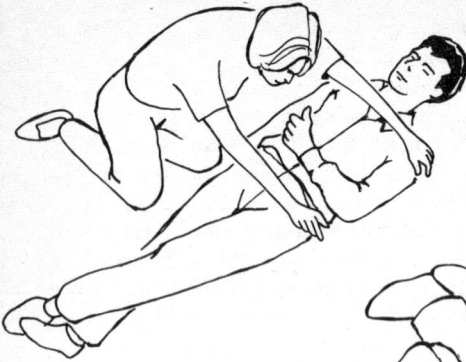

Fig. 9
Take a firm hold of the casualty's clothing with one hand, and with the other, grasp his shoulder.

Fig. 10
Gently heave the casualty towards you, so that he rests against your knees. Support his head as he rolls.

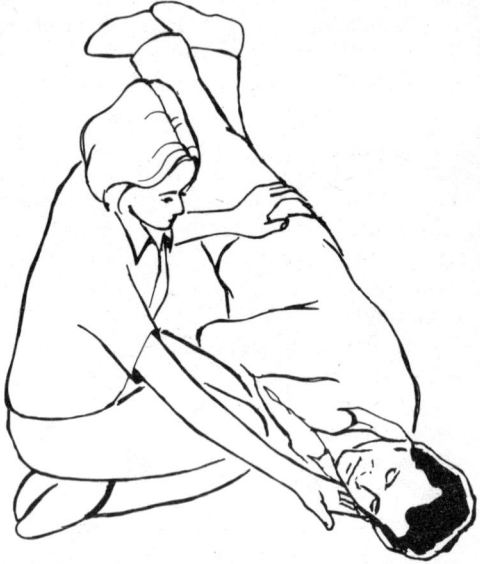

Fig. 11
Carefully move the casualty's limbs into the recovery position. Keep him in that position until help arrives.

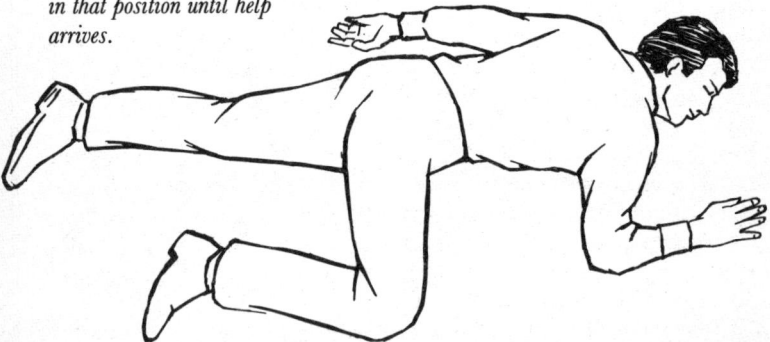

5   Check the casualty for breathing (if necessary, check again for any blockage of the airway). Tilt the head back, with the chin directed upwards and give the kiss of life twice.
6   After giving 2 breaths, give another 15 full, firm chest compressions. Check the pulse, and check it again every 3 minutes. Once it returns, stop the chest compressions immediately and continue with the kiss of life until the casualty starts to breathe naturally. Once he does, put him in the recovery position (*see below*).

If there are two of you, one should perform 5 chest compressions, followed by the other giving 1 deep breath. The person performing the kiss of life should also be responsible for checking the pulse.

☐ **Can you perform heart massage on a child?**

Yes, but the technique for babies and children is slightly different. The simple rule is lighter and faster. For children up to the age of 10, you use only the heel of one hand, and instead of some 80 compressions per minute as for adults, you perform this about 100 times per minute. For babies and very small children, the rule is lighter still and, again, faster: instead of the heel of your hand, use only 2 fingers and press down just 2–2.5 cm ($\frac{1}{2}$–1 in) at the rate of 100 compressions per minute (15 compressions should take you less than 10 seconds). As for adults, you should alternate chest compression with the kiss of life; and for all but the oldest children, you would use mouth-to-mouth-and-nose ventilation.

THE RECOVERY POSITION

Some experts say that this is the one technique that if you knew no other, you could use and still save life. The recovery position ensures that a casualty lies in such a way that the airway remains open and he cannot roll and perhaps sustain further injury.

However, if there is any reason whatsoever to suspect a back or neck injury, you should not, under any circumstances, attempt to move the casualty. You would be running the risk of inflicting permanent paralysis if you do. You should suspect the possibility of spinal damage if the casualty has suffered any violent impact.
1   With the casualty on his back, turn his head towards you, still keeping it tilted backwards with the chin pointing upwards. Remove glasses and any chunky jewelry.
2   Take the ankle furthest away from you and cross it over the other ankle.

▶ *Emergency Measures*

3 Grasp the casualty's arm that is furthest away from you. Pull it over the chest, palm downwards.

4 Now take the arm nearest you and place it under the casualty's bottom, palm uppermost.

5 You are now ready to move the casualty. Take a firm hold of the waistband or belt of the casualty's clothing with one hand and, with the other, grasp his shoulder. Gently heave him towards you. As the casualty rolls, give the head some support (figs. 9 and 10).

6 Check the position of the limbs. One arm should be bent at the elbow to keep at least half the chest from being pressed against the ground and to support the shoulder, while the other arm should extend a short distance away from the body to stabilize the casualty and prevent rolling. One leg should be bent to support the hip, while the other should be fully extended to provide stability (fig. 11).

The casualty's head should be turned to one side so that he can breathe easily. Make sure that the head is tilted back a little and that the jaw juts out, thus keeping the airway open. Remove any debris or false teeth from the mouth.

STAUNCHING SEVERE BLEEDING

Our body contains between 4–6.5 litres (7–11 pints) of blood, and we cannot survive for long if we are bleeding heavily. Blood pressure will drop, causing fainting, followed by unconsciousness and, eventually, loss of breathing and heartbeat, then death.

If the blood appears to be spurting from the body, you will know that a main artery has been cut. The main arteries in the body supply the subsidiary systems of arteries and veins all over the body.

The principle of stemming blood loss is a combination of pressure and elevation. Direct pressure should be applied to the site of the blood loss, unless the wound contains some foreign matter such as glass. In this case, direct pressure must be exerted alongside the wound.

1 Using your hand (even if it is dirty), press down on the wound immediately. Make the casualty lie down. However, do *not* move him if you think this may disturb a fracture.

2 If the casualty is losing blood from an arm or a leg, raise the limb and support it in order to reduce the blood flow in that area.

3 Cover the wound with a thick pad. If you are at home and it is readily available, cover it with a sterile dressing. If not, use any clean piece of clothing or other fabric to cover the wound. Press it to control the blood loss and encourage the natural process of blood clotting.

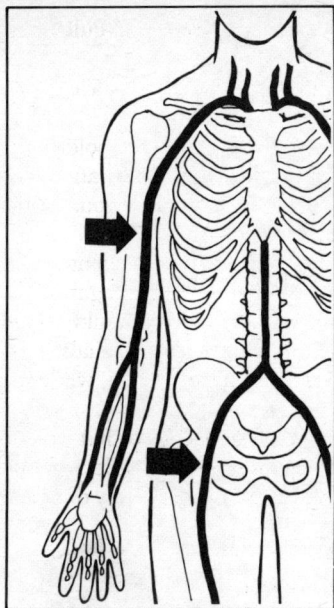

Fig. 12

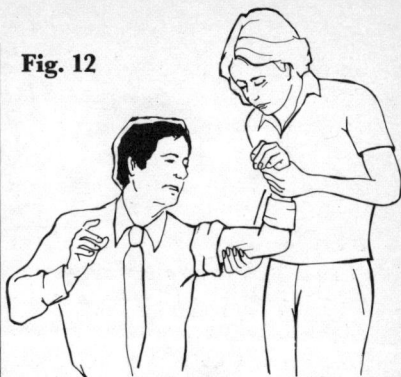

If the casualty is losing a great deal of blood from an arm wound, apply indirect pressure to the site by pressing the brachial artery.

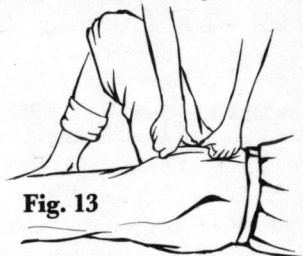

If the casualty is losing a lot of blood from a leg wound, apply indirect pressure to the site by pressing the femoral artery.

Fig. 13

▶ *Emergency Measures*

Bandage this very firmly in place, using anything to hand (e.g. necktie, tights).

4   If the wound is gaping open, try to hold the sides together and bandage quite tightly. Remember, however, that tight bandaging can be applied for only up to 15 minutes as it will effectively cut off the circulation to the entire area.

5   When bandaging is complete, summon medical help.

6   If the casualty is losing a great deal of blood and it appears to be spurting, you will have to apply indirect pressure to the site by pressing on one of the main arteries: the *brachial artery* if an arm is wounded (fig. 12), and the *femoral artery* if it is a leg (fig. 13).

7   If the casualty continues to lose blood, do not be afraid to exert more pressure. Do not exchange the dressing for a clean one; simply add another on top so that, if clotting has started to take place, you do not disturb it.

8   While waiting for help, treat for shock (*see* Chapter 3, page 25).

Fig. 14

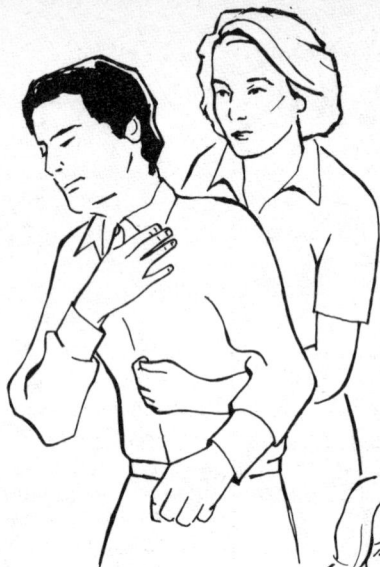

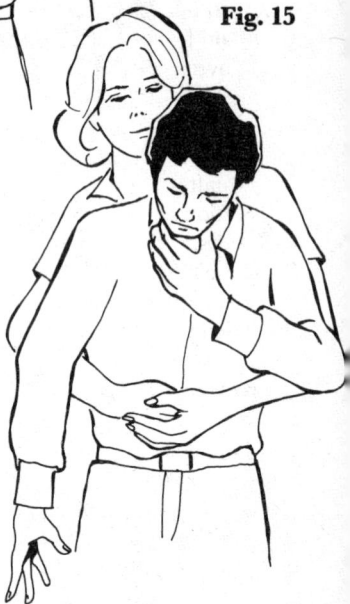

Fig. 15

To use the technique of abdominal
thrust, stand behind the casualty and put
one arm round his abdomen. Clench your
fist, with your knuckles facing outwards
(fig. 14). Place your other hand over
this fist and pull both hands quickly
towards you (fig. 15). If the casualty
becomes unconscious, lay him down and
exert a firm thrust into his abdomen with
the heel of your hand (fig. 16).

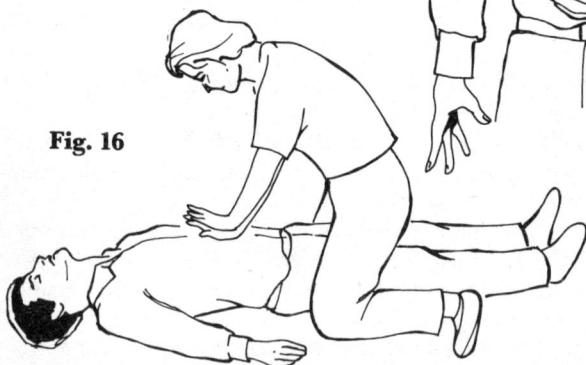

Fig. 16

ABDOMINAL THRUST
(HEIMLICH MANOEUVRE)

If someone is choking and is clearly having severe difficulty in breathing, give 4 hard blows in quick succession between the shoulder blades.

If this fails, get the casualty to bend over so that his head is lower than his lungs, and give 4 more hard blows between the shoulder blades. Repeat up to 4 times if the obstruction in the airway is not cleared.

If this fails – and only if it does – you should carry out abdominal thrusts. By using this technique, you are aiming to force air out of a choking casualty's lungs by applying thrusts to the upper abdomen. As there is a possibility of damaging internal organs, this must only be practised as a last resort.

1 Stand behind the casualty and put one arm around the abdomen just above the waist but below the ribcage. Clench your fist and place it, knuckles outwards, in the centre of the casualty's abdomen (fig. 14). Place your other hand over this fist.

2 Pull both hands quickly and firmly towards you, thus compressing the casualty's upper abdomen (fig. 15). You are trying to dislodge an obstruction in the airway, so the thrust must be quite firm. Repeat up to 3 times.

3 If the casualty becomes unconscious, lay him on the ground, face up, and place the heel of your hand on the upper abdomen, between the base of the breastbone and the navel; cover this with your other hand. Exert a firm thrust into the abdomen with an inwards and upwards movement (fig. 16). If it does not work at first, do it again up to 3 times.

4 If the thrusts do not work, revert back to 4 sharp blows between the shoulder blades; then try the thrusts again.

☐ What if a child chokes?

Treat an older child in the same way, first with blows to the back and, if that fails, with abdominal thrusts, using less pressure than you would for an adult.

Babies and small children should be placed stomach down on your lap (*see* fig. 17 *overleaf*), with head and hands pointing towards your feet. Slap between the shoulder blades 4 times, using much less pressure than you would for an adult. If this fails, lay the child on the ground and treat as for an adult, using much less pressure.

Fig. 17
To treat a choking baby or small child, place him with his stomach on your lap, and slap him 4 times between the shoulder blades.

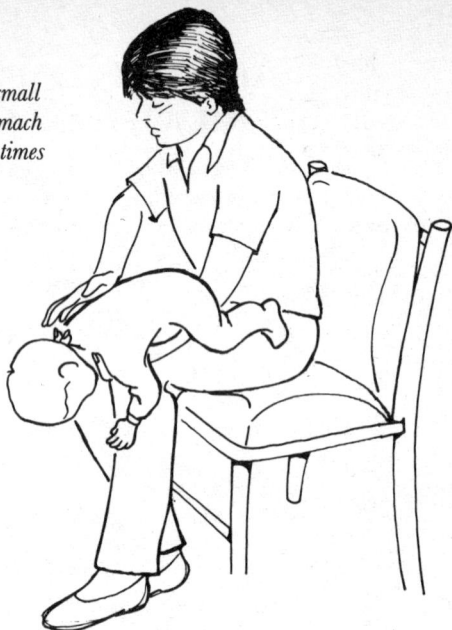

LIFE-SAVING IN WATER

Entire books and training courses have been devoted to the subject of life-saving. All that is possible here is a brief description of basic techniques. Only with correct training to an approved standard should the more dangerous rescue by direct personal contact be effected. (For details of courses, contact The Royal Life Saving Society UK, Mountbatten House, Studley, Warwickshire, England B80 7NN, Telephone 052 785 3943.)

1 The paramount consideration is the safety of the rescuer. Assess the situation carefully before taking any action.

2 Try and extend help from dry land or a boat: hand or throw the casualty any object that she can grasp – a rope, rubber ring, stick, ladder, oar, even your arm if you can do so safely.

3 Only enter the water yourself if there is no other means of helping the victim, and never do so in dangerous conditions when there is a real risk of two fatalities rather than one. If you can, wade out, or take a floating aid with you – a block of wood, fishing float, or rubber ring for example.

4 Some accidents require immediate action – for instance unconscious victims or small children. Even so, without adequate training, you are likely to endanger yourself too.

5 Open water is always cold, and a rescuer will lose a great deal of body heat. There may be currents and other dangers which you cannot see from the land.

☐ Types of victim and suggested rescue procedures

1 A conscious but weak swimmer. Such a victim will respond to calm instructions and can often be rescued by throwing a buoyant aid, or by swimming out to accompany and encourage without direct physical contact. Tell them to float and conserve energy.

2 A conscious non-swimmer. This type of victim will often panic, which can be extremely dangerous for the rescuer. Use all land-based forms of rescue if possible. Offer reassurance, but avoid direct physical contact as the victim may clutch you in panic. If you have to enter the water, swim out with a buoyant support or a strap or rope for towing the victim.

3 An unconscious victim. Such casualties will need immediate contact rescue, but this can only be safely carried out with proper training. A strong swimmer may effect a rescue using backstroke. With the victim to one side, place your arm beneath and round their body to hold the chin above water.

Fig. 18

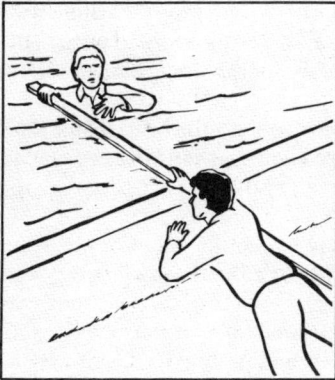

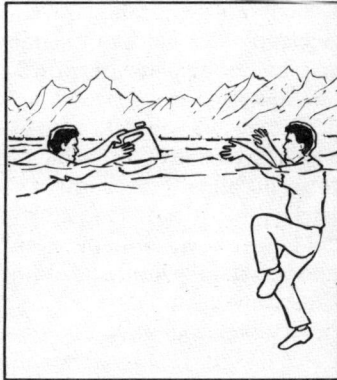

Reach out from the land with an object for the victim to grasp and pull on. Hold on to something sturdy yourself.

Swim out with a buoyant aid and accompany the victim back to land.

☐ **Once on dry land**

Once you have got the casualty back on dry land, remember the ABC of saving life and act immediately:

A *for airway*   Is it obstructed? If so, clear it.

B *for breathing*   Look for the rise and fall of chest and abdomen. Can you feel her breath on your cheek? If she is not breathing, start the kiss of life straightaway.

C *for circulation*   Can you hear the heartbeat when you put your ear to the chest? Can you feel the pulse either at wrist or neck? If not, alternate chest compressions with the kiss of life.

Finally, get the casualty to hospital. Anyone who has been rescued from drowning must receive qualified medical care for shock, for hypothermia and/or for water congestion of the lungs, the evidence of which may not be apparent for some hours.

ALTERNATIVE METHOD OF ARTIFICIAL RESPIRATION

If it is impossible to give the kiss of life, because of facial injuries or a jaw fracture for instance, this is an alternative but less efficient method of getting a casualty to breathe. Do not use this method of artifical respiration if there are arm or chest injuries, unless there is no alternative.

1   Lay the casualty down on his stomach. Turn the head to one side. Place the casualty's arms above his head with the hands placed one on top of the other. Turn the head to one side so that one cheek rests on the hands.

2   Place one hand on the casualty's head and the other on the chin, and position the head so that it is tilted back and the jaw juts out with the mouth open (fig. 19).

3   Position yourself at the casualty's head so that you are looking down the length of his back; assume a semi-kneeling position with one knee by the casualty's head and the foot of your other leg just outside the angle of his elbow.

4   Put your hands just below the casualty's shoulder blades, with your thumbs close to the spine. Rock forward and, with the power of your

Fig. 19

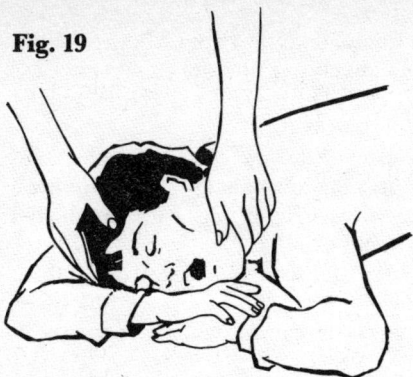

Place the casualty on his stomach with his arms above his head. Turn the head to one side and tilt it back so the jaw juts out with the mouth open.

Fig. 20

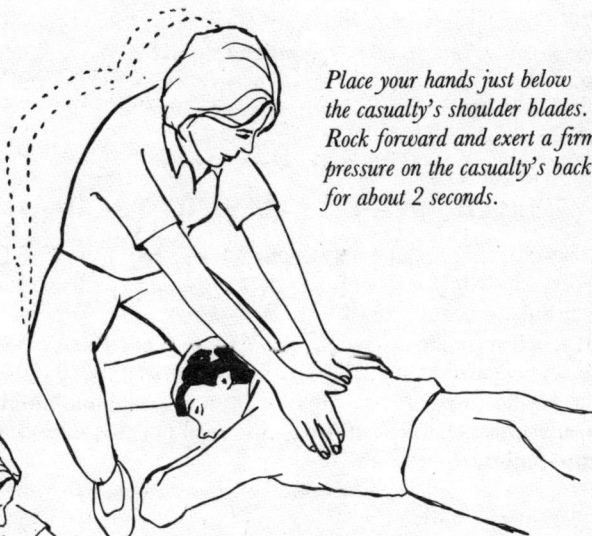

Place your hands just below the casualty's shoulder blades. Rock forward and exert a firm pressure on the casualty's back for about 2 seconds.

▶ *Emergency Measures*

Fig. 21

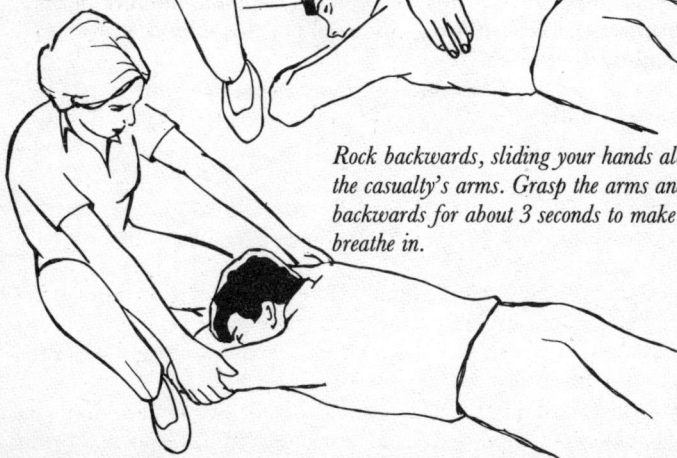

Rock backwards, sliding your hands along the casualty's arms. Grasp the arms and pull backwards for about 3 seconds to make him breathe in.

body extending through your arms and keeping your elbows straight, use your weight to exert a firm but not heavy pressure on the casualty's back for about 2 seconds (fig. 20). This should make the casualty breathe out.

5 Allow your body to rock backwards to your original position and, as you do so, slide your hands up along the casualty's arms until you reach the elbows. Now grasp the arms and pull backwards for about 3 seconds in order to make him breathe in (fig. 21).

6 Now lower the casualty's arms and slide your hands down them until you reach the back, as before, with thumbs close to the spine. Repeat the sequence, designed to encourage the casualty to breathe in and out, about 12 times a minute, allowing about 2 seconds for breathing out and 3 seconds for breathing in.

7 You may have to do this for some time and you will probably find it exhausting, but do not be tempted to think that it is doing no good – this technique has been known to save many lives even in seemingly hopeless situations. Watch the casualty carefully all the time for the first sign of unaided breathing.

LEARNING LIFE-SAVING TECHNIQUES

These techniques, correctly applied, have saved many, many lives, and everyone should feel confident of being able to perform them. St John Ambulance and the British Red Cross both provide courses of instruction in life-saving techniques and first aid, and this is the best way to learn how to do them and to practise them. Check the telephone directory for the address and telephone number of your nearest branch; alternatively, your local police station will be able to give you their address.

PART II

FIRST AID
A–Z

ASPHYXIA

This is a potentially fatal condition in which there is insufficient oxygen in the blood, as a result of either restricted breathing or inhaling smoke or poisonous fumes such as those from carbon monoxide emitted from car exhausts or those from smouldering foam-filled upholstery.

□ **Action**

1 Do not imperil your own life; this will not help the casualty. Try to separate the cause of asphyxia from the casualty, either by dragging the casualty away from the source, by throwing open windows and doors or by turning the car engine off.

2 The casualty may come round as soon as she receives fresh air if the cause of asphyxia was the result of inhaling poisonous fumes. If not, or if the cause was restricted breathing, clear the airway, and prepare to resuscitate with the kiss of life and chest compressions (*see* Chapter 4, pages 30–35).

See also Asthma Attack; Winding.

ASTHMA ATTACK

When someone is clearly having great difficulty in breathing and is wheezing audibly, you should suspect an asthma attack.

Three people in every 100 suffer from chronic, lifelong asthma, and most of them are allergic to something in their environment, such as feathers (in pillows and cushions), the fur of domestic cats and dogs, house dust mites (which live on household dust) or pollen.

If someone with no previous history of asthma has an attack, particularly while they have been asleep or lying down, you should suspect cardiac asthma, which is associated with heart failure rather than classic asthma. You should call 999 and prepare to resuscitate if necessary. Also remember that gasping for breath may be a sign of shock (*see* page 25).

☐ **Action**

Have the person sit up in order to minimize the pressure on the chest muscles and lungs. Better still, have him sit astride a chair, facing its back, and rest his arms on the chair back. This posture helps to lift the weight of the body from the chest. If he is in bed, give him support with pillows. Encourage the casualty to breathe slowly from the abdomen, *not* the chest. Talk to him calmly and reassuringly – panic will make things worse.

Either ask the casualty or search his pockets or bag for an inhaler or broncholilator and encourage him to use this. If the breathing fails to improve, call for a doctor at once, informing him or her of the nature of the problem. If the casualty starts to turn blue (around the lips first), call 999 and give the kiss of life and chest compressions if the heart stops (*see* Chapter 4, pages 30–35).

BACK INJURIES

These injuries can be caused by falls and awkward movements – such as simultaneously twisting and stretching or stretching and lifting – and, in older people, can be the consequence of the bones becoming more brittle and the discs less springy. Over 2 million people in Great Britain have to consult a doctor each year for back pain: although some have chronic back conditions, many injuries are simply the result of demanding too much of the back.

☐ **Action**

DO NOT MOVE ANYONE WHO HAS A SUSPECTED BACK INJURY. If you do, you may cause further injury to the spinal column which could result in permanent paralysis. First check whether the casualty can move at all. If she can, it is more likely that a muscle, ligament or disc has been injured rather than that the spine itself has been damaged.

If the casualty is capable of movement, get her to lie flat on the floor, cover her to keep her warm and call for a doctor. If you are outside, get the casualty into a car if possible and take her to hospital; if this is not feasible, keep her warm and call for an ambulance.

If the casualty cannot move, simply make sure she is warm and call for an ambulance, telling them that it is a back injury.

☐ How can I prevent them?

If you are predisposed to back injury, do not ask too much of your back. Never attempt to lift, push or pull anything that you know is really too heavy for you to manage: ask someone to help. If you want to pick up something, bend at the knees rather than the waist. If you are intending to do some physical activity that you do not do regularly – e.g. gardening – do not do it for too long at one stretch. You should also try to vary the activities so that you do, say, a little digging, a little weeding and a little pruning in rotation. After a week of working at a desk, do not attempt several hours digging at the weekend. Your back muscles will rebel.

● Make sure that working surfaces are at the correct height for you, and that your seat is at the correct height in relation to the working surface.
● Do not bend or stretch when ironing.
● Use a pair of steps to reach into high cupboards or change light bulbs.
● If you work at a desk, make sure that the seat is high enough for you to be 'on top of the task' – the golden rule for back sufferers. If your feet do not touch the ground comfortably, place them on a small stool beneath the desk.
● In a car, make sure the seat is in the most comfortable position for you, you can reach the foot controls easily and you can see in both mirrors without having to stretch.

BITES AND STINGS

All bites and stings are potentially dangerous: a dog can make a nasty wound (and, in certain countries, could be carrying rabies); jellyfish and other exotic creatures living in the sea are capable of injecting poisons into your skin; parrots and cats can produce unpleasant infected wounds; and some people are allergic to bee stings and will therefore require treatment.

☐ Dog bites

If the skin is not broken, there is no need to worry. If the skin is punctured, you should treat the wound (*see* Cuts and Wounds).

▶ *First Aid A–Z*

Obtain medical assistance for any large wounds.

If the bite occurs in a country where rabies is present, go to the nearest hospital casualty department. Qualified medical assistance is required immediately to determine the possibility of rabies and the appropriate treatment. If possible, try to ensure that the authorities are notified so that the offending dog can be captured and examined.

☐ **Bee and wasp stings**

Remember that a bee usually only stings if worried or annoyed. However, a wasp may sting for no reason at all. If a wasp comes near you, always keep as still as possible, particularly if you are in a confined area. Waving your arms about and trying to swat these insects with a newspaper often does you more harm than them.

Sometimes stings can't be avoided. If possible, try to remove the sting with a pair of sterilized tweezers. Bathe the area with antiseptic lotion. Apply a cold compress (ice cubes wrapped in a clean dressing) to relieve pain and reduce the swelling.

If anyone is stung by a swarm of bees or wasps, call 999 immediately. The casualty may go into anaphylactic shock, the symptoms of which are: nausea, constriction in the chest, difficulty in breathing, sneezing and facial swelling (especially around the eyes), rapid pulse, vomiting (sometimes), and eventual unconsciousness. (Treat as for traumatic shock – *see* page 25.)

Those who are allergic to bee stings may develop such symptoms from just one sting. Emergency medical treatment is essential.

☐ **Bites from small insects**

Small insects such as mosquitos, midges, ants and fleas will bite, but usually, in this country at least, they are not very dangerous. Treat mosquito bites with antihistamine cream – and do not scratch them or they may become infected.

If you discover flea bites or you suspect that your cat or dog has fleas:

1   Treat the pet with a spray obtained from your vet.
2   Treat carpets, other soft furnishings and your pet's bedding with a special flea spray, also available from your vet.
3   Remember to treat your pet again 2 weeks later (or according to the vet's instructions) in order to kill off any new fleas resulting from eggs laid in the animal's coat.
4   Avoid flea bites by spraying your pet regularly in the summer.

☐ **Snake bites**

Try to calm the casualty first and remind her that, in Britain, there is only one poisonous snake: the adder. Its bite is only rarely fatal.

● Do *not* bandage or bind the wound.
● Do not try to suck out the poison.

Encourage the casualty to keep still, explaining that the poison will circulate more quickly around the body if she moves around. Wash the wound thoroughly, and immobilize it as for a broken bone. Keep the casualty warm: shock (*see* Chapter 3, page 25) may make her cold and faint. Obtain medical assistance from the nearest casualty department as soon as possible, or call for an ambulance if you have no other form of transport.

☐ **Jellyfish stings**

These are very painful but most are not actually dangerous. Calamine lotion will relieve the stinging. If the sting is near the neck or mouth, watch carefully for any swelling that might cause the patient to stop breathing, and see a doctor if the pain or swelling continues into the following day.

☐ **Sea urchin stings**

These unpleasant sea creatures have spines to protect themselves against enemies, including humans. If you step on them, the spines break off in your foot and can be extremely painful. Although it may feel like a bite, it is not; the spines must be removed, however, and the wounds thoroughly disinfected.

If possible, carry the casualty in order to prevent any pressure being exerted upon the soles of the feet and get them to the nearest casualty department. If this is not feasible immediately, remove as many of the spines as you can with sterilized tweezers, wash the affected area and bathe with antiseptic solution.

☐ **Bites from parrots and other cage birds**

Birds' beaks contain many germs and a wound can easily be infected. Wash thoroughly and bathe with antiseptic lotion; then apply a sterile dressing (*see* Cuts and Wounds). Consult a doctor the following day if the wound appears not to be healing or if it looks infected with yellow pus around the site.

▶ *First Aid A–Z*

There is also a rare form of pneumonia (*psittacosis*) that is caused by an infection carried by birds of the parrot family. If a casualty begins to feel generally unwell a week or so after a bite, consult a doctor.

BLEEDING

If someone is bleeding heavily, refer to Chapter 4, pages 36–37, and dial 999 for an ambulance.

If the casualty is not bleeding so heavily as to constitute an emergency, you should be able to staunch it yourself. Only call the emergency services if the cause or site of the wound warrants it (*see below*). Follow the instructions for staunching bleeding given in Chapter 4, pages 36–37.

☐ The head

Bleeding may be copious if there is a head or scalp injury and you will be hampered in your treatment by the presence of the casualty's hair. Do not press on the wound – there may be a fracture underneath. Apply a dressing larger than the wound, bandage this in place (figs. 22 and 23) and take the casualty to hospital.

☐ Nosebleed

If a head injury is suspected, call for an ambulance immediately. Sit the casualty down and get her to drop her head forward. After making sure that she is breathing through her mouth, have her squeeze the soft fleshy area at the sides of the nose to help clot the blood. Make sure that she sits quite still and does not talk, cough or sniff. After 10 minutes, she can release her nose and check that the bleeding has stopped. If it has not, continue for up to half an hour. If it has not stopped by then, the casualty should see a doctor or the emergency department of the nearest hospital. Once a nosebleed has stopped, the sufferer should not blow her nose for some hours afterwards.

☐ Internal bleeding

If someone passes blood either in urine or faeces (which can appear either bloody or black and tarry), they should see a doctor without delay: this is a symptom of something seriously wrong. The same applies if blood is coughed up or vomited.

Fig. 22

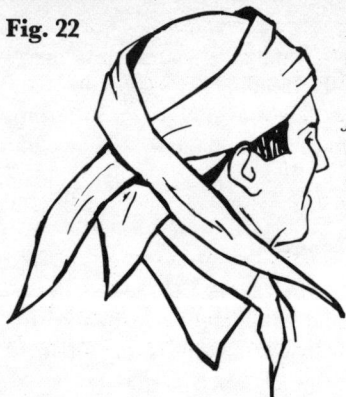

After you have applied the dressing, fix it in place with a large triangular bandage. Turn over the top of the longest side to form a hem. Place this side on the head with the points of the bandage hanging down at the back of the neck.

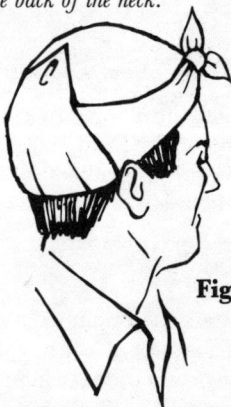

Cross over the long ends, bring them round to the front and tie in a reef knot on the forehead. Turn up the point and pin in place.

Fig. 23

If a woman bleeds very much more heavily than usual, either at the time of the usual monthly period or at a different time of the month, or she bleeds heavily for more days than usual, she should consult her doctor.

If a pregnant woman starts to bleed even slightly before the estimated time of delivery, she should consult her doctor at once (*see* Miscarriage).

Lastly, should a woman bleed vaginally, even lightly and intermittently, between periods, she should consult her doctor.

☐ The mouth

This can be severe and, in any case, hospital treatment should be sought in case stitches are required. In the meantime, have the casualty staunch the bleeding by pressing on the wound or, ideally, by pressing on a sterile dressing that covers the wound.

☐ The ear

This is a serious symptom for which the casualty must have hospital treatment. It could signify a perforated eardrum or fracture of the base of the skull.

□ **The palm of the hand**

This can produce a great deal of blood. Immediately apply pressure to the wound and raise the arm. When the bleeding begins to stop, place a thick pad (a thick sterile dressing if this is available) on the palm; have the casualty make a fist over this, and bandage the whole hand firmly.

□ **Deep chest and abdominal wounds**

Immediate hospital treatment is the priority here. Lay the casualty on his back with head and shoulders raised. Staunch the bleeding with a sterile dressing en route or while you wait for an ambulance. Prepare to give resuscitation as described in Chapter 4, pages 30–35.

BLISTER

This is a minor ailment which is best left alone to heal itself. Once a blister is pierced, the raw skin beneath can easily become infected and, in any case, will take longer to heal than if the blistered skin had been left intact.

If the blister opens up or you think it might become damaged, cover it with a sterile dressing (*see* Cuts and Wounds). Remove the dressing at night so that the skin has a chance to breathe and heal. Apply a sterile dressing the following morning for protection if necessary.

BROKEN (FRACTURED) BONES

You should always suspect a fracture after a heavy or awkward fall or a collision – for example, on the rugby field, on the ski slopes or in a traffic accident.

□ **Action**

Unless it is absolutely necessary to remove a casualty from a situation that may cause further damage (e.g. a busy motorway), do not move a casualty that you suspect may have fractured a bone. This is particularly true if you suspect a back or neck injury. By moving them, you risk causing further damage to the spine which could result in permanent paralysis.

If it is the ankle or leg that is injured and it is necessary to move the casualty, position yourself at her good side, have her put her arm across your shoulders and hop/hobble as gently and carefully as possible. The

Fig. 24
For a lower leg fracture, place soft
padding between the knees and ankles,
and then bandage the two legs
together.

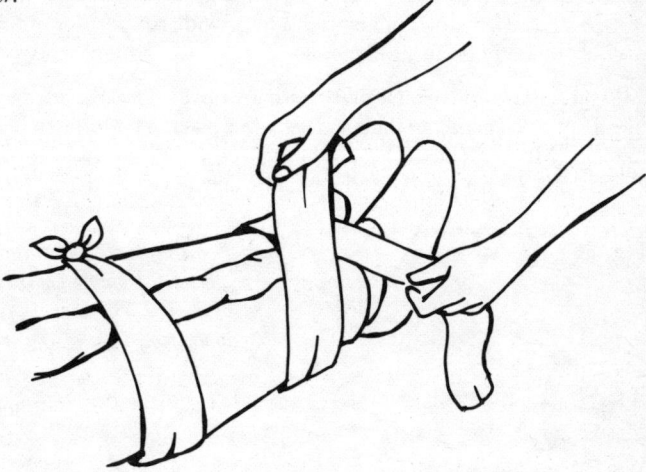

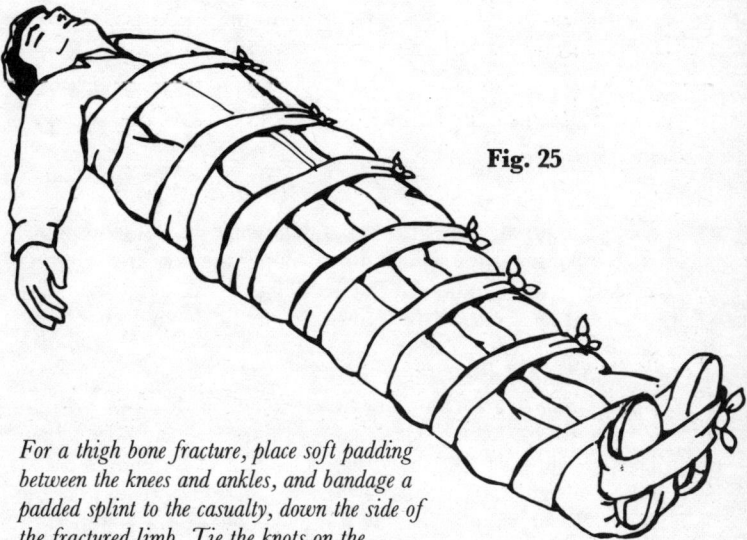

Fig. 25

For a thigh bone fracture, place soft padding
between the knees and ankles, and bandage a
padded splint to the casualty, down the side of
the fractured limb. Tie the knots on the
uninjured side.

casualty should not put weight on the injured leg. Try to remove the shoe and sock/tights.

Make sure that the casualty is warm – use your own clothing to cover her if nothing else is available – and seek qualified medical assistance urgently.

One of the principles of first aid is to provide support for an injured part of the body by using the good side.

● If you have to move a casualty with a suspected *leg fracture*, bandage the affected leg firmly to the good leg, after placing padding in between the legs. Move the good leg to the injured leg to do this. *See* figs. 24, 25, 26 and 27 for support bandaging of suspected leg and foot fractures.

Fig. 26

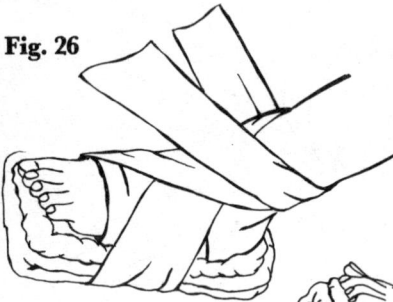

For a suspected foot fracture, place soft padding under the sole of the foot. Bandage the padding to the foot.

To secure the bandage, cross the ends around the ankle and then over the front again. Knot under the foot. This provides support until the casualty can receive medical help.

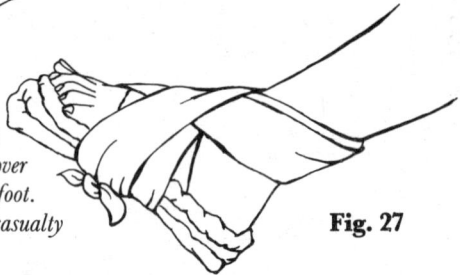

Fig. 27

● If the *arm* is injured, use either a bandage or article of clothing to make a temporary supporting sling. Slope the forearm slightly upwards and tie the bandage at the neck (figs. 28 and 29).

● For suspected *pelvic fracture*, have the casualty lie down on her back. She may be more comfortable with some support (e.g. a blanket, clothing) under her knees.

● *Collar-bone fractures* are commonly caused by putting out an outstretched arm to break a fall. Use a sling, or improvise one with a belt, tie or jersey, to support the elbow (figs. 30–32). If it is the right collar bone, take the right hand towards the left shoulder and support the right elbow. Reverse the procedure if the left collar bone is injured.

See also Bruising; Concussion; Dislocation; Falls; Paralysis.

Fig. 28
For an arm injury, you should use a triangular bandage: place one point at the neck the same side as the injured arm.

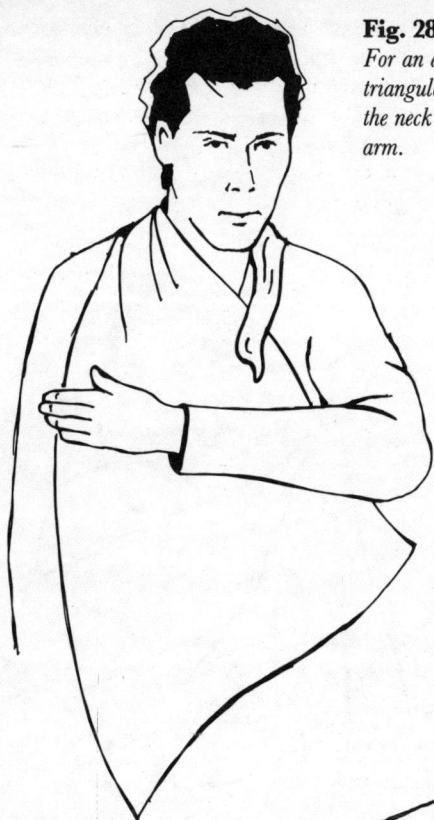

Fig. 29
Take the bandage around as shown, enveloping the arm and tie the points in a reef knot. Secure the elbow point of the bandage with a safety pin.

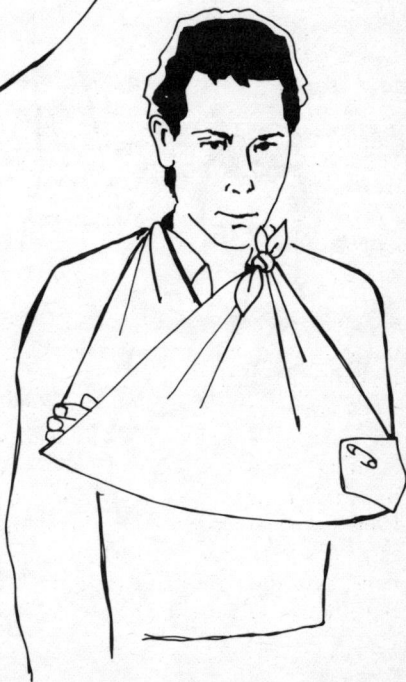

Fig. 30

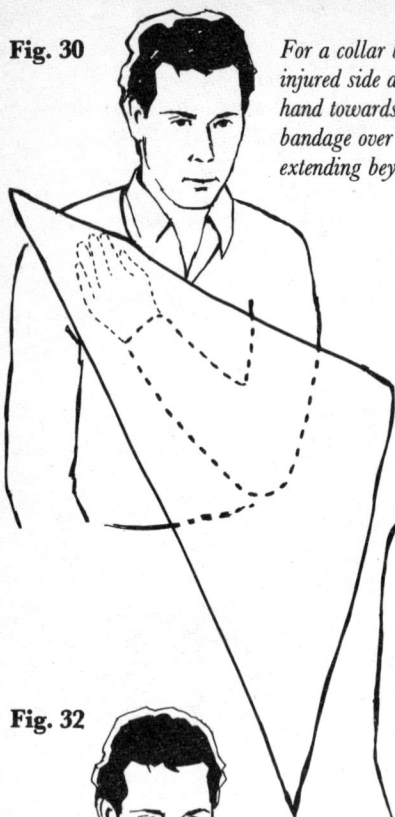

For a collar bone fracture, position the arm of the injured side against the casualty's chest, with the hand towards the shoulder. Place a triangular bandage over the hand and arm, with the point extending beyond the elbow.

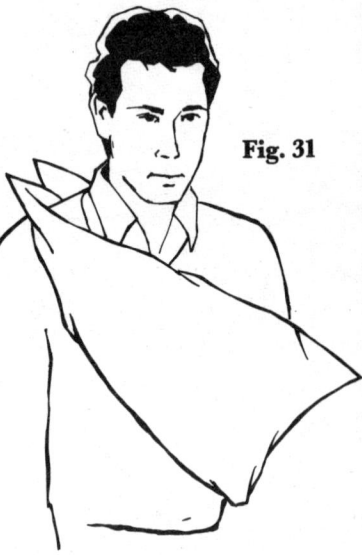

Fig. 31

Fig. 32

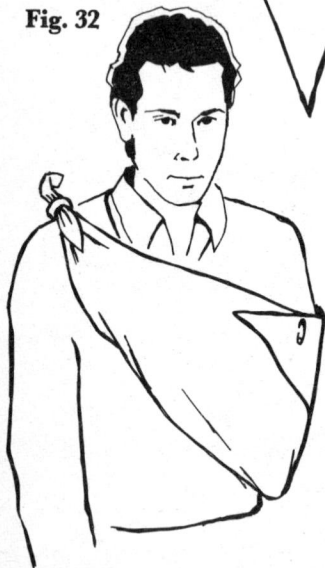

Gather the long side of the bandage from the good side of the body around the injured elbow and forearm; take the point around the casualty's back.

Tie the two ends of the bandage together at the uninjured shoulder. Tuck in the loose end at the elbow and secure with a safety pin.

BRUISING

A bruise is caused by bleeding under the skin often due to a fall or to a blow to the surface of the body. Minor bruises are nothing to worry about. Large bluish-purplish bruises, accompanied by swelling, can be treated with a cold compress to reduce swelling and relieve pain. In the case of any extensive and painful bruising, you should consider the possibility of more serious injury.

See also Broken (Fractured) Bones.

BURNS AND SCALDS

First aid can give the casualty immediate relief and minimize the injury.

☐ Types of burns

Burns fall into various categories, practically all of which could be avoided if care is taken over home safety.

Dry burns are caused by any form of fire – e.g. lighted cigarettes, hot irons and hobs, bonfires and hot barbecue coals. Sunburn (*see separate entry*) is also a dry burn.

Wet burns, commonly known as scalds, are caused by boiling water, steam (notably from kettles and uncovered saucepans of boiling water) and sizzling cooking fat.

Chemical burns include those caused by common household products such as bleach, ammonia, oven cleaners and caustic soda (all of which you should use rubber gloves to handle) and from outdoor products, notably wood treatments for wet and dry rot and general preservatives (again, rubber gloves must be used). When not being used, do ensure that these products are kept on a shelf or in a cupboard, well out of the way of inquisitive young children.

Cold burns are caused when the skin is in contact with ice-cold metal. This most frequently happens if you grasp a metal ice cube tray from the refrigerator. Hold it lightly at the edges instead.

Friction burns are a result of contact with a revolving brush (as used on floor polishers) or a moving rope or wire.

Electrical burns are caused by contact with a live electric wire or lightning (*see* Electric shock).

▲ *First Aid A–Z*

☐ **Action**

1 Bathe the affected area under slow-running cold water, or immerse it, for at least 10 minutes. Burns damage and weaken the skin so do not turn the tap on fully. Cooling the skin as quickly as possible reduces the pain and swelling, and also helps to prevent damage to the tissues beneath the skin, as well as shock.

2 Do *not* apply anything other than water to the affected area: no lotions, ointments or grease. Do *not* touch or otherwise interfere with the burned area.

3 Remove any constricting articles such as clothing and jewelry, which may be difficult to remove later if the swelling increases.

4 Because the skin has been damaged, burns are particularly susceptible to infection, so cover the affected area with a sterile dressing. If it is available, use a sterile dressing that is made from a non-fluffy material, such as a newly washed sheet or pillow case, to avoid the risk of lint or fluff landing on the burn. Never dress a burn with an adhesive plaster. Do not break blisters or remove any loose skin from the injured area. Lightly bandage the sterile dressing in place (you want air to circulate over the burn to help healing).

5 Give the casualty frequent sips of water and, if necessary, treat for shock (*see* Chapter 3, page 25).

6 A doctor should be consulted for any burn larger than a 2p piece. If the burns are extensive or cover more than about 10 per cent of the body, seek hospital treatment immediately so that the casualty may be treated for infection and shock.

See also Asphyxia.

CHILDBIRTH

If someone is obviously in an advanced state of pregnancy and is experiencing regular and frequent contractions, you may be sure that she has started labour. Nine times out of 10 you will have time to call for an ambulance or drive her to the hospital where she has made arrangements to have the baby. If you do call for an ambulance, be sure to tell them that the woman has started to give birth, and how often the contractions are coming.

If, however, the contractions are coming every couple of minutes, the baby may start to emerge at any minute. Do *not* go for help: give help on the spot. Never abandon a woman who is actually giving birth. Your help could save life.

☐ **Action**

Ideally, you should have ready:

● a plastic or rubber sheet to lay beneath the mother
● towels
● a flannel and a bowl of warm water (to wipe the mother's face)
● string and scissors
● boiling water (to sterilize the string and scissors)
● sterile dressings
● something warm with which to cover the mother and the baby – e.g. a soft blanket, towel or even a clean jersey

It does not matter what position the mother adopts when giving birth. It may be more convenient for you if she lies down, but she may be more comfortable in a squatting position. Make sure that she is free of clothing from the waist down and talk to her quietly and reassuringly. Don't panic if she screams a lot and appears to be in agony: childbirth is normally quite a painful experience.

All this time, the mother has been experiencing regular contractions, and her waters may have broken. After a while, she will begin pushing to expel the baby. Once the head appears, you must tell her to stop pushing; instead, she should pant so that it does not emerge too quickly. Support the baby's head, without exerting any pressure upon it. If there is a translucent membrane covering the baby's face, tear it away gently with your fingers.

Now check whether the umbilical cord can be seen or felt around the baby's neck. If it is, gently loop it over the baby's head or shoulder, reminding the mother to pant, not push, as you do so. If the cord remains around the baby's neck as he is born, he may be strangled.

The baby's head will turn to one side and you should continue to support it with both hands while waiting for the baby's shoulders to appear. As they do, hold the baby beneath the arms and gently lift him as he comes out of the mother's body.

Place him on the mother's belly, stomach down with the face turned to one side. Do not pull on the umbilical cord. You will notice that the cord is pulsating: this has been the baby's lifeline while he has been in the womb; through it, he has been fed fluids and nutrients via the placenta.

With some clean fabric remove any blood and mucus from the baby's mouth. The baby may cry within a minute or so – do not worry if he does for this is a good sign. You only need to worry if the baby does not make a sound, appears not to be breathing or turns blue. After you lay the baby on the mother's belly, cover them both in something warm – your own clothing if there is nothing else available – and make sure that the baby's face turns outwards so that the airway is free.

Shortly after the birth, the mother will feel renewed contractions; this signifies the delivery of the afterbirth (placenta), which is attached to the cord. Do not attempt to pull on the afterbirth and do not cut the cord. Allow the afterbirth to be expelled freely and then place it near the baby so that the cord does not come under any strain. Place a cloth or sanitary towel on the mother's vulva to catch any discharge.

Once the cord has stopped pulsating, and if you have sterilized string and scissors, you can detach the placenta and cord from the baby. You should tie the cord firmly in 2 places with pieces of sterilized string – one about 20 cm (8 in) and the other about 15 cm (6 in) from the baby – and cut the cord between these two ties. If you have a sterile dressing, place it over the cut end of the cord.

After about 10 or 15 minutes, check the cord beneath the dressing to make sure that it is not bleeding. Provided that the string is tied tightly enough around the cord, there should not be any. If there is, tie another piece of string quite firmly around the cord – do not remove the original piece.

Regardless of whether you have had to deal with any bleeding, you should now tie a further piece of string around the cord about 10 cm (4 in) from the baby's abdomen.

Use a second sterile dressing, if available, to cover the cord. Lay the cord on the baby's abdomen and secure it with a bandage or a towel around the baby's body. If you do not have a sterile dressing, leave the cord exposed to the air: this will be very much more hygienic than any piece of fabric other than a sterile dressing (newborn babies are particularly vulnerable to germs).

Retain the cord and placenta for later examination in hospital; a doctor or midwife will need to make sure that everything is as it should be – for example, that nothing has been left inside the mother's body that should have been expelled.

If you do not have sterilized string and scissors available, or feel less than confident about cutting the umbilical cord, then there is no need to do so. Leave it until qualified medical staff arrive. Simply keep the afterbirth and cord near the baby, and keep the baby warm.

☐ **What to do if mother or baby starts to turn blue**

Attend to the mother first and give the kiss of life. Then help the baby. Check that the airway is clear, by carefully wiping the baby's nose and mouth. If the baby still does not breathe, give a mouth-to-mouth-and-nose resuscitation. (*See* Chapter 4, pages 30–32.)

CHILL (HYPOTHERMIA)

The most important principle in the treatment of excessively low body temperature – known as *hypothermia* – is to restore the casualty's body temperature to normal at roughly the same rate that it reached the abnormal level. If someone has become severely chilled in response to a chilly environment, therefore, they should be warmed slowly by heating their environment. If, on the other hand, they have become suddenly chilled, as they would if they were plunged into an ice-cold sea, they should be warmed up rapidly.

☐ **Action**

If the casualty is shivering, hypothermia will only be at an early stage. Shivering is the body's way of trying to heat itself. Provide a warm environment for the casualty and offer warm drinks.

If the casualty's temperature is under 95°F (35°C), and she is pale, lifeless and freezing cold to the touch, with a slow pulse and breathing rate, you may assume that hypothermia has set in. (*See also* page 25 for further symptoms in adults.) If the casualty is in an advanced stage of hypothermia, she will not be shivering and this, coupled with a subnormal temperature, should make you suspect hypothermia immediately. However, a baby with hypothermia often looks rosy, rather than pale, and the only symptoms may be low body temperature, slow pulse and breathing and general lethargy.

Provide a warm environment with heating, blankets and hot water bottles (wrapped in towels and placed on the chest in order to raise the body's core temperature rather than that of the limbs). Hold a baby next to your skin and wrap yourself and the baby in a blanket. Seek urgent medical assistance as this is a serious condition in which the internal organs can be severely damaged.

Never use an electric blanket: this will cause blood to rush to the skin surface, away from the vital organs. For the same reason, *never* give alcohol.

☐ **How to prevent it**

People vary in what they regard as the ideal temperature for their home environment, but it should not fall below 63–68°F (17–20°C) for

▲ *First Aid A–Z*

those who are sedentary and especially the elderly and infants.

Wool, cotton or thermolactyl underwear is essential for cold, wintry conditions. The extremities should be protected as well, with socks, or heavy tights, lined boots, gloves and a warm hat – some 90 per cent of the body's heat is lost from the head.

See also Frostbite.

CHOKING

This can develop within a minute or two into a life-threatening situation for which emergency action is the only situation. Refer to Chapter 4, page 39.

See also Asphyxia; Hiccups; Winding.

CONCUSSION

If there has been any sort of serious head injury, you should suspect concussion, and in all cases, the casualty should receive qualified medical treatment.

Concussion is, literally, a violent shaking or disturbance of the brain within the skull. The casualty may lose consciousness temporarily, and have a pale face, clammy skin, a fast but weak pulse and shallow breathing. He may either feel nauseous or vomit, sometimes an hour or so after the accident.

Loss of memory (amnesia) of the events occurring just before and just after the accident is a reliable pointer. If, however, the casualty cannot remember events that occurred several hours before and/or after the incident, a more serious injury is indicated.

☐ **Action**

1 Check casualty for any other injuries.
2 Place casualty in the recovery position (*see* Chapter 4, page 35.)
3 Arrange urgent removal to hospital.
4 Monitor breathing rate and pulse while you await the arrival of ambulance, and be prepared to resuscitate if necessary.

CONVULSION (SEIZURE, 'FIT')

This involuntary contracting and relaxing of the muscles is a symptom of irritation of the brain. The two most common causes are high fevers in children, when the convulsions are called *febrile fits*, and epilepsy (*see* Epileptic Seizure).

☐ **Febrile fits**

1 Ensure that the room is well ventilated.
2 Remove or loosen any constricting clothing.
3 If the child becomes unconscious, check the ABC of resuscitation (*see* Chapter 4, page 29).
4 Sponge the casualty's skin with tepid water to bring down the temperature.
5 Consult a doctor without delay.

If a child has a series of fits without regaining consciousness, emergency medical treatment must be sought immediately.

See also Poisoning.

CRAMP

There are several different categories of this painful and spasmodic contraction that can occur in some muscles of the body and there are a variety of causes.

☐ **Night cramp**

If you should wake in the night with cramp in your leg or foot, first try to stretch the limb as much as possible and rub it both for warmth and to increase blood flow to the affected muscle. Make sure the bedroom is sufficiently warm and well ventilated. If you suffer chronic night cramp, consult your doctor.

☐ **Stomach cramp**

This usually indicates a gastric disorder, but it can also accompany painful menstruation. If it is the latter, taking Codeine or Veganin may ease the pain. If it persists, a doctor should be consulted.

☐ **Swimmer's cramp**

This usually results from swimming in water that is so cold that the muscles involuntarily contract, thus making it impossible to swim any further; or from swimming for too long, with the same result. In addition, if you have eaten less than an hour before swimming, much of

▶ *First Aid A–Z*

your blood will be attracted to your digestive organs, away from your limbs, thus making cramp more likely. The casualty must be warmed as rapidly as possible, and the ABC of life-saving techniques administered if necessary (*see* Chapter 4, page 29).

☐ **Heat cramp**

If you exercise in excessive heat, you will sweat a great deal. This can result in the loss of an excessive amount of fluid, salt and other vital minerals, and as a consequence, cramp will occur. As a remedy, make the casualty drink as much water as possible; add $\frac{1}{2}$ teaspoon of salt to every pint (0.5 litre) of water.

☐ **Functional cramp**

People whose work demands that they use one part of the body for many hours at a time may experience cramp in the over-used part. Writers and musicians are particularly prone to this. Unfortunately, no remedy been discovered. It used to be thought that this sort of cramp was hysterical in origin and caused by an unconscious desire not to do the particular activity. This was unfair to these sufferers as it is now known that such cramps are a symptom of a genuine brain disease which affects those parts of the brain that control fine muscular activity. Ask your GP to refer you to a neurologist.

See also Convulsion; Epileptic Seizure.

CUTS AND WOUNDS

Minor cuts and wounds will probably bleed for only a short time. If the bleeding is severe, refer to Chapter 4, pages 36–37.

☐ **Action for minor cuts and wounds**

1   Wash the area thoroughly with slow-running warm water. Wash your own hands before you attempt to treat and dress the wound.
2   Once the bleeding has stopped, make sure that the wound is completely clean. If it is a surface graze, it is likely to contain dirt and debris which must be removed, and the area must be thoroughly cleansed and treated with antiseptic lotion.
3   If the wound contains any foreign matter, such as splinters or pieces of glass, try to remove it with a pair of sterilized tweezers if

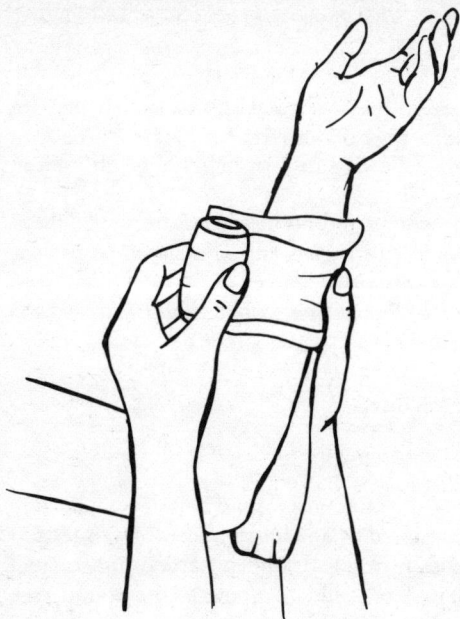

Fig. 33
Open the folded sterile dressing without touching the surface. Place it gauze-side down over the wound.

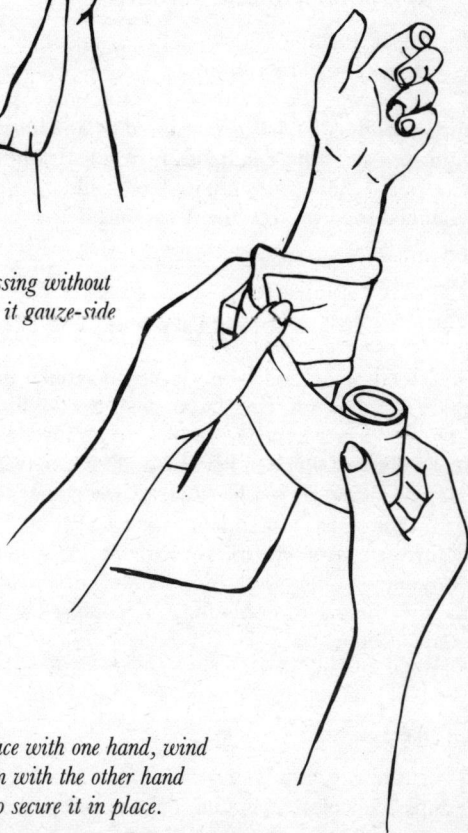

Fig. 34
Holding the dressing in place with one hand, wind the bandage around the arm with the other hand and fix with a safety pin to secure it in place.

possible. Do not attempt this if you think there is a risk of pushing the foreign matter further into the wound; instead, seek emergency medical treatment.

4 Once the cut or wound has been cleansed and treated, it may be dressed with a sterile dressing (figs. 33 and 34).

5 Change the dressing the following day, or before this if it is clear that the dressing is already soiled.

6 Take a good look at the wound and the discarded dressing: if there is any sign of pus, the wound is infected and you should consult a doctor or attend the nearest casualty department.

7 Any wound that refuses to close always requires hospital treatment in case stitches are required. This is especially true of facial cuts.

☐ **Action for puncture wounds**

1 Wash the area as thoroughly as possible for several minutes.

2 Do *not* dress the wound.

3 Determine the nature of the puncture wound before you take any further action: if it has been caused by an animal bite, refer to Bites and Stings; if it is the result of an accident with a garden fork or nail outdoors, where contaminated soil could have entered the wound, seek qualified medical treatment without delay.

See also Bites and Stings; Bleeding.

DIABETIC CRISIS

A diabetic who mistakenly takes too much insulin, misses a meal or takes so much exercise that a great deal of his blood sugar is used up may develop a hypoglycaemic ('hypo') reaction – that is, he has too low a level of sugar in his blood. This can lead to diabetic crisis, and may be followed by a life-threatening coma. If you know the casualty to be diabetic, you should suspect diabetic crisis if he exhibits the following symptoms: dizziness; drowsiness; weak, rapid pulse; profuse sweating; shallow breathing; confusion and disorientation. Unfortunately, these symptoms may be confused with drunkenness. If you come upon a stranger with these symptoms, search him for a card or medallion, which all diabetics carry with them.

☐ **Action**

1 If the casualty is conscious, give sugar immediately – e.g. sugar lumps, chocolate, biscuits, cakes, sweets, honey. If the casualty is suffering from too little insulin (*hyperglycaemia*), this amount of sugar will not affect the outcome.

2 If the casualty fails to improve within a few minutes of taking sugar, he is more likely to be suffering from hyperglycaemia and needs less sugar, not more. Arrange urgent removal to hospital unless you can get the casualty to take insulin in the normal way.

3 If the casualty is already unconscious, do *not* under any circumstances attempt to feed him sugar as this could result in choking. Place him in the recovery position (*see* Chapter 4, pages 35), and arrange his urgent removal to hospital. Be prepared to resuscitate if he stops breathing (*see* Chapter 4, pages 30–35).

DIARRHOEA

Sudden and acute diarrhoea can be caused by eating something that does not agree with you, as well as food poisoning, anxiety or (in women) a monthly period. Food poisoning is often accompanied by nausea and/or vomiting, stomach cramps and pain, and medical treatment is required. Consult your GP if acute diarrhoea persists for more than a day and continue taking plenty of fluids.

Chronic (i.e. long-lasting) diarrhoea can be caused by lesions of the small intestine, certain diseases of the colon, anxiety or some gastro-intestinal operations. In any event, you should consult your GP.

☐ **Action**

1 Drink plenty of fluids in order to make up the body's losses and prevent dehydration.

2 For the time being, avoid alcohol, coffee, aspirin, cigarettes, hot and/or spicy food, raw vegetables and wholemeal foods, notably bread, muesli, bran cereals and other bran products.

3 Seek medical advice if the diarrhoea persists.

☐ **Diarrhoea in babies and small children**

Sudden or chronic diarrhoea in babies and young children can be life-threatening as they can become dehydrated extremely quickly. You should seek medical assistance without delay. In the meantime, give the child as much liquid as possible, adding $\frac{1}{2}$ teaspoon of salt and 1 teaspoon of sugar to every pint (0·5 litre) of water, to replace that lost by the body. Do *not* give paediatric kaolin mixture.

See also Indigestion.

▶ *First Aid A–Z*

DISLOCATION

This is the displacement of one or more bones at a joint. The joints most frequently dislocated are those of the shoulders, elbows, thumbs, fingers and lower jaw. It is also possible to dislocate the hips and the knees. The joint appears deformed and will be very painful. When a joint has received such a severe impact as to dislocate it, it may also be fractured and should therefore be treated as such (*see* Broken [Fractured] Bones).

☐ Action

1 Arrange for the casualty to be removed to hospital immediately.
2 Make sure that the casualty is warm and, if possible, made comfortable and supported with cushions.
3 Do *not* attempt to pull bones back into place.

DROWNING

See Chapter 4, pages 42–44.

EARACHE

Earache is one of those symptoms which usually calls for medical assistance rather than first aid, especially if accompanied by impaired hearing, dizziness, fluid or blood emanating from the ear, or fever. There are, however, two exceptions: earache caused by pressure changes and earache caused by a foreign body in the ear.

☐ Earache caused by pressure change

This can occur during air travel, while driving up and down steep mountain roads or scuba diving. The sufferer should try one of the following:

● yawning
● sucking a boiled sweet
● closing the mouth, squeezing nostrils together and slowly blowing out

Babies can suffer from pressure changes, too, especially on aircraft. Always ensure that a baby is feeding during take-off and landing: the sucking will help the pressure equalize in the ears.

☐ **Foreign body in the ear**

1   Do *not* do anything if you feel that you may cause further damage – for example, if the foreign body is glass. Do *not* under any circumstances poke anything into the ear for this could in itself cause damage and could also push the foreign body in further. For anything other than an insect in the ear, the casualty should go to hospital immediately.

2   If the casualty can feel vibrations or movement within the ear, it is possible that the foreign body is an insect. Have the casualty sit down by a basin or bath and lean the head sideways and down, so that the affected ear is uppermost. Fill a jug with tepid water and pour it slowly over the ear; some of the water will enter the ear canal and the insect should float out. Do *not* do this if the ear is painful or if there is any possibility that the eardrum has been perforated.

3   If this does not work, the casualty should be taken to hospital.

ELECTRIC SHOCK

DO NOT TOUCH THE CASUALTY IF HE IS STILL GRASPING THE SOURCE OF THE ELECTRICITY. The important thing to remember is that you should remove the casualty from the source as quickly as possible, without also injuring yourself.

☐ **Electric shock from the domestic supply (low voltage)**

1   Turn off the supply if possible, either at the mains or the wall switch.

2   If this is not possible, separate the casualty from the source using something made of a *dry* material that is a poor conductor of electricity – e.g. a wooden broom or stool or a large plastic object, such as a bin. You should wear rubber boots or stand on a thick pile of newspapers. The aim is to break the electrical circuit so that it does not pass straight from the casualty's body into your own.

3   Electric shock can be enough to stop the casualty's heart and also cause extensive burns and internal damage. First, check the ABC of life-saving, and, if necessary, restore the casualty's heartbeat (*see* Chapter 4, pages 32–36).

4   Treat the casualty's burns with slow-running cold water as quickly as possible (*see* Burns and Scalds).

5   If the casualty is conscious, treat for shock (*see* Chapter 4, page 25).

6   Summon emergency medical help.

▶ *First Aid A–Z*

☐ Electric shock outdoors (high voltage)

If the casualty has suffered an electric shock outdoors, from lightning during an electrical storm, or from a high-voltage current from an electric pylon or the 'live' rail of a tube train system, the shock may cause extensive internal damage and burns, and can prove fatal.

In the case of high-voltage current, come no closer than 18m (20 yd). On no account must you touch the casualty. Call the emergency services (ambulance and fire), telling them the cause. Also call the electricity board's emergency number to have the current switched off.

In the case of a lightning strike, check the casualty's breathing and resuscitate if necessary. Also treat for shock and be sure to keep the casualty warm, covering them with your own clothes if necessary. They should receive urgent medical treatment.

EPILEPTIC SEIZURE

Most forms of epilepsy are caused by an instability of the electrical rhythms of the brain. There is usually no actual physical damage to the brain itself. The condition often runs in families. In about 1 in 5 cases, particularly when epilepsy occurs in later life, a physical cause, such as a brain tumour or a stroke, should be suspected; this should be fully investigated by a consultant neurologist.

In a typical epileptic seizure (a 'fit'), the sufferer falls to the floor, unconscious. His body becomes rigid; it is at this stage that the sufferer may bite his tongue and be incontinent. Then this stage gives way to the next, in which the muscles relax and contract rhythmically. This phase usually lasts for only a few minutes and the sufferer remains still for about 10 minutes before regaining consciousness. An epileptic seizure usually lasts about 15 minutes from beginning to end.

☐ Action

1 Do not try to restrain the casualty.
2 Remove any constricting clothing if possible, and move any furniture or other hazards to prevent injury to the sufferer.
3 When the casualty's limbs stop jerking, place him in the recovery position (*see* Chapter 4, page 35).
4 The convulsion is normally sudden and brief with the sufferer shortly regaining consciousness. If he does not, you should seek medical assistance.

5 If the sufferer sustains an injury as a result of the seizure or if the casualty has several consecutive seizures, medical treatment should be sought immediately.

6 When the casualty comes round, ask him if he has any medication and, if so, help him to take it. Suggest that he rests.

EYE INJURIES

These can be extraordinarily painful and should be treated by qualified medical staff.

☐ Burns

Burns caused either by hot substances or by corrosive, irritant chemicals should be treated immediately by bathing the eye in running water. This is a case in which first aid, promptly given, can do much to minimize pain and permanent damage. The easiest method is to get the casualty to a sink and run water from the cold tap over the eye, which should be positioned closest to the base of the basin. The good eye should be uppermost so that no contaminated water runs into it. In the case of chemicals, you may have to continue this for some time to ensure that the chemical has been sufficiently diluted.

After giving first aid, take the casualty to hospital. Be sure to tell medical staff what caused the burn, particularly in the case of irritant chemicals.

Burns to the retina (the light-sensitive layer at the back of the eye) can be caused by exposure to the sun, particularly if you look at an eclipse without protecting the eyes, and in conditions of bright sun combined with snow (*see below*).

☐ Foreign bodies

If the casualty's eye is red, painful and watering, it is possible that a foreign body has damaged the protective cornea. If the foreign matter appears to be lodged in the eye, or is adhering to the coloured part of the eye (i.e the iris and the pupil), take the casualty to hospital immediately for professional treatment. Any injury of the eyes is potentially serious, for the cornea may develop a scar which will affect the eyesight.

If a foreign body, such as an eyelash or a piece of grit, enters the eye, you should be able to wash it out. Have the casualty lean over a basin with the good eye nearest the bottom of the basin and the affected eye

▶ *First Aid A–Z*

uppermost, and pour a jug of tepid water over the eye. Alternatively, have the casualty sit on a chair and tilt the head backwards so that you can examine the eye. Wash both hands thoroughly first. Using your first finger and thumb to separate the lids, ask the casualty look up, down, right and left so that you can see what is causing the discomfort. You may be able to remove the foreign body by touching it lightly and gently with a slightly dampened, clean dressing or handkerchief.

If there is no water available, have the casualty blink repeatedly as this, together with the watering of the eye, may succeed in dislodging whatever has entered the eye.

If these efforts fail, the casualty should be taken to hospital for qualified medical treatment.

☐ Insect and animal bites

Bites in and around the eyes should be thoroughly washed with tepid running water as described above and, in almost all cases, the casualty given qualified medical treatment. The only exception to this rule would be if the injury were minor and near the eye but not in it – for example, a mosquito bite. (*See* Bites and Stings.)

☐ Snowblindness

This potentially serious condition occurs when bright sunshine is reflected off pure white snow, throwing up a dazzling glare. This can blind you for a short period, but prolonged exposure can lead to permanent damage to the eye, affecting sight.

1 Cover the eyes with dark glasses, ski goggles or whatever is to hand; pull a woollen hat further down over the eyes.

2 When you arrive indoors, bathe the eyes with cold water to alleviate redness and watering; then apply eye pads or rest in a darkened room.

3 If the condition persists into the following day or is clearly already severe, obtain medical assistance urgently. Make sure that you are seen by a qualified ophthalmologist as well as a doctor.

FAINTING

A faint is a brief lapse into unconsciousness from which the casualty usually recovers within seconds. If she does not, you should look for other causes for the loss of consciousness: make sure that the airway is clear and check breathing and heartbeat.

A brief faint, as distinct from a deep state of unconsciousness, can be caused by: a hot, poorly ventilated atmosphere; fatigue; anxiety or a nervous reaction; lack of food; blood loss; standing still for a long time.

☐ **Treatment for an impending faint**

If the person is very pale and feels dizzy, you may be able to prevent a faint by having her sit down and put her head between her knees in order to restore the blood circulation. Get her to take deep breaths and, as she does, increase the room's ventilation if you can. If she has been standing for a long time – say, at a bus stop or in a crowd – suggest that she flex her leg and foot muscles, so that the large amount of blood that normally collects in the lower body in this position has the chance to circulate more freely.

☐ **Treatment for an actual faint**

1 Make the casualty comfortable, preferably by laying her flat on the ground, face up, with the legs raised. Do not support the head with a cushion.

2 Check in pockets, wallet, handbag for a card that may indicate a condition such as diabetes or epilepsy, which may be the cause of the faint. Alternatively, the casualty may be wearing a bracelet or medallion with this information.

3 Check that the airway is clear and that the jaw and chin are directed upwards. Check the casualty's breathing and heartbeat: if either one has failed, proceed with resuscitation techniques immediately (*see* Chapter 4, pages 30–35).

4 Provided that the casualty is breathing and you can hear the heartbeat, it is likely that she will come round in a few seconds. Raise your voice a little and call her name as this may bring her round.

5 If she does not come round quickly, seek emergency medical treatment.

See also Diabetic Crisis; Epileptic Seizure; Heart Attack; Heat Exhaustion and Heatstroke.

▶ *First Aid A–Z*

FALLS

A fall is a shock to many of the systems of the body, and the extent of that shock is related to the severity of the fall. A minor fall, such as when someone trips up and falls lightly – which toddlers and small children do frequently, usually with no ill effects – is usually not serious and only reassurance and sympathy are required, with attention to any grazing (*see* Cuts and Wounds). A moderate fall, such as when someone skids on ice and lands full length upon the back, is potentially more dangerous and sometimes requires medical treatment. A severe fall – from a height, for example – will almost certainly require emergency medical treatment.

NOTE Any loss of consciousness should always be investigated.

□ **Action**

1 Reassure the casualty, especially if it is a child. For a severe fall, do not make any attempt to move the casualty until she shows that she is capable of movement herself. Be alert to the possibility of sprains and strains (*see separate entry*), dislocated joints (*see* Dislocation), fractured limbs (*see* Broken [Fractured] Bones), concussion (*see separate entry*) and head injury.

2 If she is not capable of movement but is conscious, establish which part of the body is injured. If it is a leg or arm, *see* Broken (Fractured) Bones. If it is the back, *see* Back Injuries. Do not move the casualty under any circumstances: if the spine has been injured, and the casualty is then moved, further damage may be done which could result in permanent paralysis. If the head has been injured, there may be skull fracture or concussion (*see separate entry*), and movement should be kept to a minimum. For both spinal and head injuries, keep the casualty warm, using your own clothes if necessary, and call the emergency services for an ambulance.

3 If the casualty has lost consciousness, move her into the recovery position. Carry out the ABC of life-saving and resuscitation if necessary (*see* Chapter 4, pages 29–35). Call the emergency services for an ambulance.

4 Check for any sign of bleeding and, if necessary, staunch it, ideally, with a sterile dressing. If one is not to hand, use a clean handkerchief and a piece of clothing. If the casualty is losing a lot of blood, your priority is to reduce blood loss rather than worry about hygiene. (*See* Cuts and Wounds).

5 Make sure that the casualty is kept warm to minimize the effects of shock (*see* page 25), and increase the room's ventilation if necessary.

See also Bleeding; Paralysis; Winding.

FINGERNAIL INJURIES

☐ Torn nail

If the nail is torn below the white part – i.e. into the 'quick' – trim the white part neatly with a clean pair of sharp nail scissors. Allow the nail to grow out. If needed to keep the injured area clean, wear a plaster; you should also wear rubber gloves if you immerse your hands in water. If there is any sign of infection, such as pus issuing from the area, wash thoroughly, treat with antiseptic lotion and consult your GP.

☐ Crushed nail

Blood may appear beneath the nail if it has been crushed. Run the affected finger(s) under cold running water for at least 5 minutes to stem the blood flow. Consult your GP, particularly if the finger was crushed severely, if a fracture is suspected or if there has been damage to the nail bed.

☐ Ragnails

These are the tough little pieces of dead skin and cuticle that sometimes break away from the base of the nail. They should be trimmed neatly, without going too close to the living part, and Vaseline applied in order to keep the skin supple. Cuticles should always be pushed down at bath time with the tip of a special instrument – an 'orange stick', available from any chemist – wrapped in cotton wool, in order to prevent ragnails developing.

See also Whitlow.

FISHBONE, LODGED IN MOUTH OR THROAT

This can be extremely painful. Because of the risk of infection, the bone should always be removed, rather than left in the hope that it may work itself out.

☐ Action

1 Sit the casualty on a chair and have him tilt his head backwards with the mouth wide open under a good light.
2 Using a newly sterilized pair of tweezers, take hold of the fishbone,

as closely to the surface of the mouth or throat as possible, and pull gently.

3 Once the fishbone has been removed, have the casualty wash out his mouth with an antiseptic gargle.

4 If you find that so little of the fishbone protrudes from the surface that you cannot get hold of it, or that it is too far down the throat, the casualty should be taken to hospital for its removal.

'FITS'

See Convulsions, Epileptic Seizures.

FRACTURES

See Broken (Fractured) Bones

FROSTBITE

If any of the outer parts of the body – such as the fingers or toes, nose or ears – feel numb and have turned a waxy white or bluish colour, frostbite is indicated. This is particularly true if conditions are below freezing, and the casualty has been out of doors for some time without proper protection in the form of warm gloves or mittens, warm socks and good shoes or lined boots, together with a warm covering for the head, through which is lost some 90 per cent of the body's total heat.

☐ **Action**

1 Do *not* rub with snow.

2 Remove any restrictive articles of clothing or jewelry.

3 Aim to warm the affected part of the body slowly – in other words, at the same rate that it became cold. Do not apply hot water bottles.

If the fingers are affected, take off any covering and have the casualty place them in her armpits and tell her to hug her arms close to the body.

If one of the casualty's feet is affected, remove any covering and place her foot beneath your armpit so that it may derive warmth from your body.

If the casualty's nose or ears are affected, remove your gloves and cup your hands over the affected area in order to transmit warmth into the casualty's skin.

4 Do *not* rub the area as the tissues are fragile and can be damaged.

For the same reason, do not apply direct heat in the form of hot water bottles, nor should you allow the casualty to warm the affected areas by a fire or radiator.

5   Once you have administered such first aid as you can, help the casualty to hospital for qualified medical treatment.

See also   Chill

GRAZES

See Cuts and Wounds

HEAD INJURY

Staunch any bleeding quickly (*see* Bleeding) and be alert to the possibilities of concussion (*see separate entry*) and neck injury (*see* Paralysis).

HEART ATTACK

The cause of a heart attack is nearly always a blood clot in one of the major arteries supplying the heart muscle. These are usually already clogged due to lifelong smoking, poor diet and/or high blood pressure (hypertension). A small clot is the last straw – the part of the heart muscle that was being fed by the blocked artery then dies.

Even a small area of damaged heart can set off what is known as *arrhythmia*. This means that the pumping of the heart becomes totally uncoordinated. Most people who die of a heart attack have arrhythmia, even though the bulk of their heart muscle is not damaged. However, provided that a heart attack victim is transferred very quickly to a hospital casualty department or even an ambulance with a defibrillator on board, they can be saved. Mouth-to-mouth resuscitation is therefore a temporary life-saving measure to keep the casualty going until qualified medical help is available.

☐ **Symptoms**

The typical picture of a heart attack is that the casualty first experiences severe pain in the chest (which he may mistake for acute indigestion), followed by collapse. Not all heart attacks manifest themselves so dramatically, however.

Heart attack is a general term that covers a sudden loss of heart function. The signs and symptoms may include:

▶ *First Aid A–Z*

- very severe pain at or above the centre of the chest or radiating up into the jaw or down the left arm
- dizziness
- difficulty in breathing
- pale or greyish complexion
- loss of consciousness
- cessation of breathing and heartbeat

Ironically, if someone complains of pain above the left nipple where the heart is, this is more likely to be an anxiety attack than a true heart attack.

□ **Action**

1   Call 999 for an ambulance. Check for vital signs: breathing and heartbeat. If the casualty is not breathing, begin the kiss of life. If the heart has completely stopped beating, begin chest compressions. (*See* Chapter 4, pages 32–35). Do *not* perform chest compressions on a beating heart, even if the pulse is extremely weak. Continue until help arrives.

2   If the casualty is conscious, make him as comfortable as you can without moving him. Any exertion at this point could have a crucial effect. Prop up his head and shoulders with pillows or anything else close to hand; alternatively he can be supported in a sitting position. Loosen any constricting clothing, particularly a tight collar or waistband.

3   Make sure that the casualty is kept warm, either with bedding or your own clothes if necessary.

4   It is essential not to panic in this situation, frightening though it is. Concentrate on looking after the casualty, and if he is conscious, reassure him that medical assistance will soon arrive.

See also   Asthma Attack (cardiac asthma); Fainting; Indigestion.

HEARTBURN

The sufferer experiences acidic gastric juices rising from the stomach into the oesophagus (the gullet). Offer the sufferer a glass of milk in order to neutralize the acid, and support the casualty in a half-sitting position with cushions. If heartburn occurs at night, sleeping propped up on two or three pillows usually alleviates the condition.

If the heartburn becomes chronic the sufferer should consult her GP. It is, however, common in pregnancy.

Heartburn has absolutely nothing to do with heart attack and should not be taken as a symptom of such.

HEAT EXHAUSTION AND HEAT STROKE

Both these conditions are responses to a hot and humid environment, to which the casualty is unaccustomed. Heat stroke, which is the rarer condition of the two, may occur not only as a result of a hot and humid environment but also as a complication of high temperature associated with disease when it rises to 104°F (40°C) or more. Heat stroke is the result of the body's inability to regulate its temperature through sweating. Emergency first aid is essential and medical assistance should also be sought urgently.

☐ **Heat exhaustion**

The casualty will probably have a headache and feel dizzy and nauseous; she will look pale and may faint; she may have muscle and/or stomach cramps; and her pulse will be fast.

1 If possible, remove the casualty to a cooler environment. Remember that rooms on lower floors, such as basements and cellars, are cooler than those on upper floors.

2 If the casualty is conscious, give her plenty of cold water to drink to which you have added ½ teaspoon of salt to each pint (0.5 litre). Ensure she drinks slowly, to avoid vomiting.

3 Sponge the casualty all over with tepid water (not ice cold as this will aggravate the condition).

4 Fan the casualty to hasten evaporation of the tepid water; this will speed up the effectiveness of the sponging.

5 Obtain medical assistance without delay: heat exhaustion, if untreated, can develop into the rarer condition of heat stroke, which can be fatal.

☐ **Heat stroke**

While someone with heat exhaustion will look pale with a clammy skin, a person suffering from heat stroke will appear flushed and will feel dry to the touch. The victim of heat stroke will also have a headache, feel dizzy and breathe noisily. Restlessness or confusion may lead to delirium and ultimately to unconsciousness and death if the condition is untreated.

1 Remove the casualty to a cooler environment if possible.

▲ *First Aid A–Z*

2 Wrap the casualty in a cold, wet towel or sheet and make sure that it is kept wet. Place her in the recovery position (*see* Chapter 4, page 35).

3 Sponge her face and neck with tepid water. Fan her, as described for heat exhaustion.

4 Obtain emergency medical treatment immediately for this life-threatening condition.

5 If the casualty is already unconscious, clear the airway and check her breathing and heartbeat (*see* Chapter 4). If she is not breathing, give her the kiss of life, checking from time to time that the towel you have wrapped her in is well dampened.

See also Cramp; Fainting; Sunburn.

HICCUPS

In hiccups, air is suddenly drawn into the lungs, after which there is a click (the hiccup) caused by the vocal cords closing abruptly. The spasmodic intake of air is in turn caused by irritation to the nerves surrounding the diaphragm, which causes the diaphragm to contract rapidly.

This irritating affliction almost never indicates a serious condition and is almost always a symptom of poor digestion or anxiety. If you have hiccups lasting for several days or longer, you should consult your GP.

□ **Action**

In the hope of immediate relief, try any of these traditional remedies:

● take a paper bag, cup it round your mouth so that it is airtight, and breathe in and out several times
● take a good drink of water
● take a drink of peppermint water (add a few drops of oil of peppermint to water)
● have a cup of peppermint tea
● hold your nose and close your mouth for about a minute – no longer

Do *not* stand on your head (another traditional remedy); you might sustain a more serious injury.

HYPOTHERMIA

See Chill (Hypothermia)

HYSTERIA

Before you decide that someone is hysterical, you should eliminate any genuine explanation for their strange behaviour. You can have hysterical physical symptoms – such as paralysis – or an hysterical emotional state. In either case, the person is responding to some stress in their life in an exaggerated fashion.

Hysteria is a sign of a troubled person. Minor or infrequent emotional outbursts are not serious, but hysterical physical symptoms are. The person should be referred by a GP to a consultant psychiatrist.

Common physical symptoms and signs that hysterics adopt include amnesia, paralysis, seizures ('fits'), numbness and blindness. Hysterical emotional states include shouting, yelling, crying with loud gasping sobs and often hyperventilation (rapid overbreathing).

☐ **Action**

1 As hysteria is essentially attention-seeking behaviour, the most effective thing to do is ignore it. The more attention you pay, the worse it will become.

2 The hysteric sometimes behaves so rashly that they are at risk of genuinely hurting themselves. This is unusual, however: hysterical fits tend not to occur hidden away in the bathroom, for example, but in some safe and public place. Attempt to isolate the person from onlookers. Escort the casualty to a quiet place. Do not physically force or restrain the casualty, but adopt a firm voice.

3 Hyperventilation, the process of rapid overbreathing which drives all the carbon dioxide out of the lungs, can lead to what is known as tetany. This is a temporary paralysis of the hands in which the hand muscles go into spasm. The treatment for this is to make the person rebreathe the carbon-dioxide-laden air they are expiring, by placing a paper (*not* plastic) bag over their mouth and nose for a short while.

See also   Convulsion; Diabetic Crisis; Epileptic Seizure; Heart Attack.

▶ *First Aid A–Z*

INDIGESTION

Also known as dyspepsia, indigestion includes uncomfortable rumblings in the stomach, stomach cramps (*see* Cramp), flatulence ('wind') and heartburn (*see separate entry*). It can also produce pain in the chest.

In most cases, indigestion is a consequence of dietary excess or anxiety. It is much more rare for it to be an indication of anything seriously wrong. Chronic gastro-intestinal irritation or disturbance can indicate the presence of an ulcer, a hiatus hernia, cancer of the stomach; and acute indigestion with a searing pain in the chest can signify a heart attack (*see separate entry*).

If, as is more likely, the indigestion has been caused by dietary excess, it will pass. Common causes of indigestion are:

- eating rich and/or spicy food
- eating contaminated food
- drinking a lot of alcohol before eating
- eating a heavy meal late in the evening
- eating a huge meal after not having eaten for a long period
- eating too quickly

Sufferers of chronic indigestion caused by anxiety or emotional upset may show a number of other symptoms as well as those of indigestion: loss of appetite/compulsive eating, sweating, palpitations and insomnia.

☐ **Action**

1 Rest. Your stomach already has too much to cope with and your digestive system is protesting. Movement or exercise places a further demand on the body.
2 Drink only fluids for a day or so, then graduate to light bland meals until you feel fit again.
3 If the indigestion is very acute and painful, or if it seems to be a permanent condition, consult your GP.
4 Peppermint tea sometimes relieves indigestion, as may the medicinal preparations designed to alleviate the condition (available from chemists). It is desirable, however, to establish the cause of indigestion and eliminate that, before treating yourself in this way.

MISCARRIAGE

If a woman starts to miscarry – that is, she starts to bleed and may feel cramping like period pains (possibly accompanied by low back pain) before the approximate date that she is expected to give birth – have her lie or sit down and rest. If the bleeding is very minor, with just a little spotting of blood, a few days' rest may prevent miscarriage. The GP should attend straightaway in any case.

If the bleeding is moderate to severe, call 999 for an ambulance: do not attempt to drive the woman yourself.

If the woman realizes that she may miscarry, she may become very distressed. Try to calm and reassure her, and urge her to be as calm as possible.

If the woman does miscarry, it will be useful if you can give the hospital anything that has been discharged from the vagina; it will be examined to make sure that nothing has been left inside, and tests may be performed on it to discover a possible cause for the miscarriage. The woman should be taken to hospital, where she will be examined. She will also need a great deal of emotional support.

MOLES, DAMAGED OR ENLARGED

Small moles are, in themselves, quite harmless, provided that they are not bruised or knocked, they do not bleed and they do not start to spread.

If the mole is bleeding, staunch it by applying a sterile dressing to the area, fixing it in place with an adhesive bandage. Consult your GP if the mole has been bleeding, if it has been severely knocked or if it starts to spread.

MOUTH ULCERS

These are small painful red areas within the mouth, usually occurring in ones and twos and lasting no longer than a fortnight. If they last longer or occur frequently, you should consult your GP. Although mouth ulcers are normally quite harmless, they can be a symptom of several more serious conditions.

□ **Action**

1 If you have just one or two mouth ulcers, cleanse the mouth morning and evening with an antiseptic mouthwash and make sure that your toothbrush is spotlessly clean. Brush the teeth after each meal.
2 Apply a strong astringent such as iodine tincture to the area every few days, and at other times, protect and soothe the area with occasional applications of honey of borax or borax glycerine (available from your chemist). Alternatively, apply bicarbonate of soda twice a day, once in the morning and once in the evening, to the affected area.
3 Avoid acid foods such as citrus fruits and tomatoes which may aggravate the condition.

▶ *First Aid A–Z*

NECK INJURY

DO NOT MOVE THE CASUALTY UNDER ANY CIRCUMSTANCES. Staunch any bleeding on the spot (*see* Bleeding) and refer to Broken (Fractured) Bones, Paralysis and Whiplash.

NOSEBLEED
See Bleeding

PARALYSIS

DO NOT ATTEMPT TO MOVE THE CASUALTY UNTIL YOU HAVE DETERMINED THE CAUSE OF THE PARALYSIS. There are several different sorts of paralysis, and finding out which muscles are involved will give you an immediate clue as to the cause.

The commonest cause of sudden paralysis is a stroke, when the muscles of the limbs on one side of the body, together with the facial muscles on that side, become paralysed. The other side of the body will be normal. Another possible cause of paralysis is damage to the spinal cord. In this case, both legs will be paralysed or if the damage is at the top of the spine in the neck, both the arms and the legs will be paralysed, but not the face.

☐ Stroke

Check that the casualty is still breathing and that you can feel the heartbeat. If not, do the ABC and the kiss of life (*see* page 30). Place the casualty in the recovery position making sure that she is kept warm, either with a blanket or with your own clothes if necessary. Obtain medical assistance immediately so that the casualty may be safely removed to hospital.

☐ Spinal damage

Do not move the casualty under any circumstances when spinal damage is suspected. Any damage could be worsened by movement, and this could lead to permanent paralysis. Make sure that the casualty is kept warm, as above, and then call 999 for an ambulance.

☐ Bell's palsy

This is a rather disfiguring facial paralysis, for which there is no appropriate first aid. Medical assistance should be sought without delay for diagnosis and the appropriate medication.

See also Falls; Hysteria.

POISONING

DO NOT ATTEMPT TO MAKE THE CASUALTY VOMIT UNTIL YOU KNOW WHAT THE POISON IS. Vomiting the poisonous substance back up the gullet can double the damage in the case of corrosive poisons. If the casualty spontaneously vomits, keep some of the vomit as this will provide the hospital's emergency department with useful clues.

☐ How can I be sure that it is poisoning?

Poisons can be swallowed, but they can also be absorbed through the skin or inhaled (as in the case of car exhaust fumes). It cannot be assumed, therefore, that if the casualty has not swallowed something, they have not been poisoned. A poison, such as a wood perservative treatment, may have been spilt on the skin and entered the body in that way. The signs to look for are:

Corrosive poisons Lips, mouth and throat may be painful and swollen. In the case of large doses, collapse and death can follow quickly.

Irritant poisons Stomach cramps and vomiting.

Narcotico-irritants Abdominal pain and vomiting as above and, in addition, confusion and convulsions, ending in stupor and death.

Whatever the cause, poisoning can lead to unconsciousness and action has to be taken quickly.

☐ Action

1 Call 999 for an ambulance. Explain that the case is suspected poisoning.
2 If the casualty is unconscious, check breathing and heart rate and, if necessary, carry out emergency procedures outlined in Chapter 4. Look round to see if there is any sign of what he may have taken, and hand it to the ambulance crew when they arrive.
3 If you are absolutely certain that you know what the poison was, telephone the National Poisons Information Service on 01-407 7600 for their advice while you await an ambulance.

▶ *First Aid A–Z*

4 If you are certain that the poison is an acid, give the casualty a glass of milk in order to neutralize the acid and minimize damage to the internal organs. Do *not* make the person vomit.

See Chapter 1, table of poisons, pages 16–17.

SCALDS

See Burns and Scalds.

SHOCK

See Chapter 3, page 25.

SNOWBLINDNESS

See Eye Injuries

SPASM, MUSCULAR

A muscular spasm is, by definition, involuntary, and it may be painful or it may not. General spasms, involving the whole body and combined with unconsciousness, are regarded as convulsions (*see separate entry*). A painful spasm that usually affects the leg but sometimes the arm is known as cramp (*see separate entry*). When the stomach, bowel or other part of the digestive tract is subject to involuntary spasm, this is known as colic. Rapid twitches, such as sometimes occur in the eye, are a minor affliction requiring only reassurance.

See also Epileptic Seizure; Hysteria.

SPLINTER

A splinter, although an apparently small and trivial injury, can infect the finger or other part of the body if it is not removed promptly. Glass and metal splinters should be removed by a doctor; wood splinters can be removed as follows.

☐ **Action**

1 If the site is dirty, have the casualty wash it very carefully with soap and water. Wash your own hands thoroughly in soap and water.

2 Sterilize a pair of tweezers and a needle in a match flame.

3 Positioning the tweezers as close to the surface of the skin as possible, try to grip the splinter. If you can, pull it out of the skin slowly and carefully. The casualty should thoroughly wash the affected site afterwards and apply antiseptic lotion.

4 If you are unable to remove the splinter in this way, or you can see that part of it is still embedded in the skin, take the sterilized needle and break the skin at the site. Use the tip of the needle to prise out the remaining piece of the splinter, and pick it up with the tweezers. Have the casualty wash the site as above and treat with antiseptic lotion.

5 If, however, you are still unsuccessful, the casualty should see a doctor in order to have the splinter removed and the area thoroughly cleaned.

6 If, after successful removal of the splinter, the affected area becomes red and swollen after a day or two, and perhaps pus can also be seen, the casualty must visit a doctor for professional treatment.

SPRAINS AND STRAINS

It is important to distinguish either a sprain or a strain from a fracture (*see* Broken [Fractured] Bones). A *sprain* occurs when the ligaments holding the bones of a joint together are either stretched or torn. Severe sprains can affect ankles, wrists and, less often, elbows, knees and shoulders; the symptoms are pain and swelling and some loss of movement in the affected area. A *strain*, on the other hand, is an over-stretched or torn muscle in any part of the body; symptoms are stiffness, cramp in the affected area, pain and swelling. If the injury appears severe – i.e. the casualty is clearly in a great deal of pain, swelling is extensive and there is a significant loss of movement – it may, in fact, be a fracture and the casualty should be removed to hospital for an X-ray.

▶ *First Aid A–Z*

☐ **Action**

1 Once you are sure that you are treating either a sprain or a strain, and *not* a fracture, follow the St John Ambulance advice:

☐ R for rest
☐ I for ice
☐ C for compression
☐ E for elevation

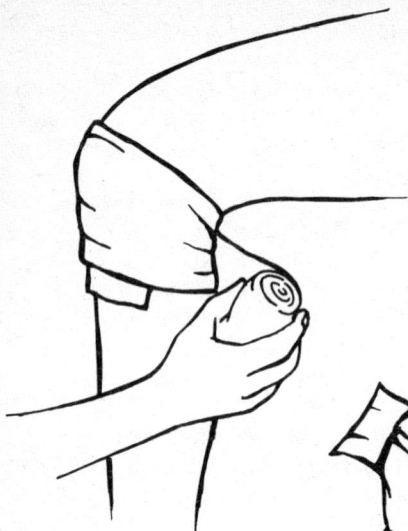

Fig. 35
When bandaging a knee, start from below the knee, then bandage straight across the knee itself.

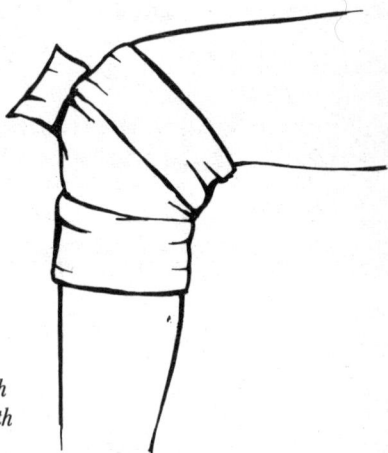

Fig. 36
Bind the bandage above and below the knee alternately, overlapping each turn. Fix the end of the bandage with a safety pin.

2   For a wrist, elbow or shoulder injury, casualties should sit on a chair. For ankle or knee injury, they should lie down, and remove shoes and socks or tights – swelling will probably continue and it may then be impossible to remove shoes and socks without considerable discomfort.

3   Apply an ice pack or cold compress to the site of the injury for at least 30 minutes to alleviate pain and to reduce swelling. (This slows the blood flow to the area.) Make sure that the casualty is otherwise warm and comfortable, and offer a cup of tea or other warm drink.

4   After about 30 minutes or so, bandage the joint (see figs. 35–38) to give some support. Bandaging is important not only for the support it gives, taking some of the pressure off the area, but also to remind the casualty of the injury so that he remembers not to over-use the joint in

For a sprained ankle,
bandage it firmly with a
stretch bandage to give
some support. Take the
bandage around the ankle
and then cross it over and
under the foot.

Fig. 37

Fig. 38
Secure the bandage by
fixing the end neatly with a
safety pin.

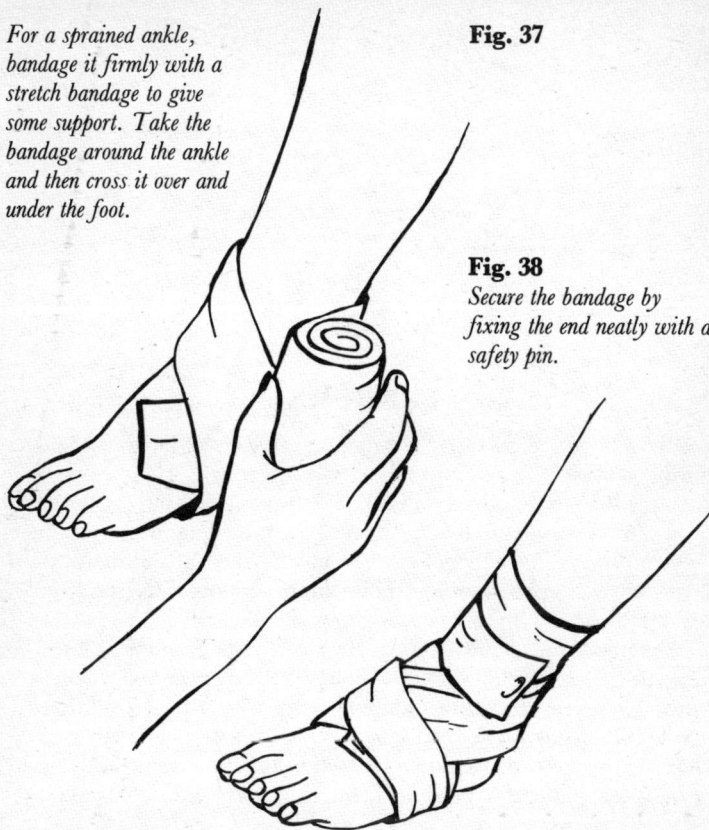

▶ *First Aid A–Z*

the days to come while it is healing.

5   The affected joint should, if possible, be elevated. In the case of an ankle or knee injury, the casualty should rest as much as possible with the leg raised, and not place weight on the affected leg until both pain and swelling have subsided. In the case of a wrist, elbow or shoulder injury, the area should be supported in a sling (*see* Broken [Fractured] Bones) and movement restricted to a minimum. The casualty should not attempt to carry any heavy weights or to drive until both pain and swelling have subsided and movement has returned.

6   Pain and swelling are to be expected with a sprain or strain, but reassess the situation the following day and observe the degree of swelling. If any doubt persists as to whether the injury is actually a fracture, consult a doctor.

STOMACH ACHE

See Indigestion

STRAINS

See Sprains and Strains

STROKE

See Paralysis

SUNBURN

Sunburn is caused by the ultraviolet rays of the sun burning the skin during prolonged exposure.

In the short term, severe sunburn can be equivalent to third-degree burns and is very painful and disfiguring. In the long term, you have only to observe the effect of the sun plus the absence of moisture in desert areas to appreciate how powerful the action of the sun can be: consider how much more delicate your skin is.

Prolonged and repeated exposure to a strong sun is known to increase the risk of skin cancer. About 1 in 1500 people develop skin cancer each year, but of this number, some 90 per cent can be cured provided that the cancer is spotted and treated early enough.

Sun protection cream should be used before sunbathing and should be re-applied after every swim. If your skin starts to feel dry or taut or looks reddened, move out of the sun or cover yourself.

In cases of moderate-to-severe sunburn, you should be alert to the possibility of heat exhaustion or heat stroke (*see separate entry*), both of which should be treated immediately and the burn given second priority.

Provided that there are no complicating symptoms and signs, such as headache, dizziness, nausea or cramps which can signify heat exhaustion or heat stroke, treat mild-to-moderate sunburn as follows. (Severe sunburn, in which the skin is bright red and blistered must be treated in hospital and without delay.)

☐ **Action**

1 Remove the casualty to a cool environment if possible. Remember that basements and ground-floor rooms are cooler than rooms on upper floors. If you cannot immediately provide a cooler environment for the casualty, try and get her into the shade (under a tree or beach umbrella, close to a car or hut, for example).

2   Remove clothing from near the affected area, gently and carefully. The casualty may be in considerable discomfort, and you should avoid rubbing the skin in any way. Having been burned, it is fragile and dried out and therefore vulnerable.

3   Repeatedly sponge the casualty gently all over with nearly cold water.

4   Give her sips of tepid water at frequent intervals.

5   After sponging, dry the skin gently and apply an oily calamine lotion or any after-sun product, to feed and moisturize the skin.

6   Fan the casualty either with a fan, a folded newspaper or a hairdryer or fan heater switched to the cold setting.

7   If you observe any blistering, obtain medical assistance without delay. Remain alert, too, to the possibilities of heat exhaustion and heat stroke, both of which are serious conditions requiring qualified medical treatment.

If you do inadvertently become sunburned, you should not expose that area of your body to the sun until it has completely healed and the skin loses any red colour. If a part of your skin that has been exposed to the sun's rays develops a rash of small moles or freckles, which do not disappear during the winter, you should not expose that part to strong sunlight again. If you are in any doubt about the condition of your skin, ask your GP to refer you to a consultant dermatologist.

TOENAILS, INGROWING OR DAMAGED

One of the most common minor disorders to be seen in hospital casualty departments is ingrowing toenail, which can be extremely painful and should be treated by a doctor or, if in its early stages, a chiropodist. Ingrowing toenails are frequently caused by cutting down the edges of the nail at the sides, so this should be avoided: toenails should always be cut straight across. They should also be kept clean to prevent debris lodging beneath the skin and causing infection.

Damaged or crushed toenails should be treated in the same way as damaged fingernails (*see separate entry*).

TOOTHACHE

First aid for toothache can only be a temporary measure because there is always an underlying cause for this type of pain. The casualty should

▲ *First Aid A–Z*

make an appointment with a dentist as soon as possible; if it appears to be an emergency – there is a lot of pain or swelling or a tooth is broken or damaged, for example – the casualty should be seen the same day. If this is impossible, and the casualty is certain that it is an emergency, contact the local hospital for details of the emergency dental service.

In the meantime, the pain can sometimes be alleviated by taking aspirin or paracetamol, and by swabbing the tooth, or the cavity, with oil of cloves or sucking a clove.

VOMITING

Being sick can be caused by a large number of accidents and diseases, and the cause should be thoroughly investigated after the casualty has been made comfortable.

□ Initial action

1 Have the casualty sit or lie down, and support his head and back with pillows.
2 Once he has stopped vomiting, take the casualty's temperature and pulse.
3 Sponge the casualty's face with lukewarm water and give him sips of cold water to wash out his mouth.
4 No further action can be taken until you establish the cause of vomiting.

□ What causes it?

Vomiting can be caused by a number of conditions, which would require a doctor's diagnosis, and by any of the following:

● Food poisoning or other poisoning (*see* Poisoning and the list of poisonous items on pages 16–17).
● Gastro-intestinal virus.
● Pregnancy, especially during the first three months and sometimes during the entire term.
● Epileptic seizure and other types of convulsions (*see* Epileptic Seizure; Convulsions).
● Concussion (*see separate entry*) and other head injury.
● Allergic reaction to a sting or bite (*see* Bites and Stings), a drug or other substance.

□ **Further action**

If you cannot identify the cause of vomiting, you should consult your GP.

If vomiting occurs more than twice in a day *or* is combined with any of the following signs, medical attention is required urgently:

● head injury
● poisoning
● allergic reaction to a sting or bite, a drug or other substance
● diarrhoea
● prolonged stomach pain
● in the case of a child, a temperature higher than 100°F (37.8°C)
● the appearance of blood in the vomit (look not only for a reddish substance but also reddish-black or black)

WHIPLASH

This injury to the neck usually occurs when someone drives into the car in which you are sitting. The collision causes your head to be violently thrown forward and immediately violently thrown back again. There may be damage to the muscles or ligaments, as in a sprain or strain, and, in rare cases, the vertebrae in the neck may be damaged or broken.

If in any doubt about a casualty's condition, do not attempt to move her if she appears to be unable to do so. The spinal cord in the neck may be further damaged and this could lead to permanent paralysis. In this situation, it is advisable to wait for the arrival of an ambulance, in the meantime keeping the casualty warm.

Even if the injury to the neck appears to be confined to whiplash, the casualty will nevertheless have to attend hospital for X-ray, treatment for possible shock and for a surgical collar which may have to be worn for some weeks.

WHITLOW

This is an acute inflammation either at the root of the nail, on the soft part of the fingertip or in the tendon coverings along the fingers, either palm side or upper side. A whitlow is a type of abscess and requires professional medical treatment. If there is any unavoidable delay in consulting your GP, a hospital casualty department should attend to it. In the meantime, cleanse with antiseptic lotion and dress with a sterile dressing.

▲ *First Aid A–Z*

WINDING

A heavy fall or a substantial blow in the lower chest just below the bottom of the breastbone – i.e. the solar plexus – can cause winding, in which the casualty is barely able to breathe and may be temporarily unable to speak. He may also be bent double with the pain, which, in severe cases, can lead either to nausea or actual vomiting.

☐ **Action**

1   Have the casualty sit down, and if possible, support the arms so that some of the weight of the body is taken off the chest.

2   Loosen a tight collar and/or waistband, and then gently rub the affected area.

3   If the casualty is unconscious (although this would be very unusual if the casualty were only winded), make sure that the airway is clear, check for signs of breathing and make sure that you can feel the pulse. Prepare to resuscitate if necessary (*see* Chapter 4, pages 30–35). If the casualty does not regain consciousness in less than a minute, you should assume that winding is either not the correct diagnosis or is not solely responsible for the casualty's condition.

See also   Asthma Attack; Bites and Stings; Choking; Heart Attack; Paralysis.

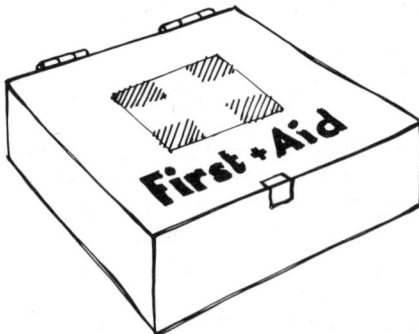

INDEX